Running High, Running Low, Running Long

To prove to my daughter anything was possible I ran to the start of my next ultra marathon. And then ran it.

Ben Rolfe

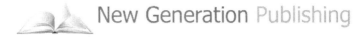

New Generation Publishing

For Jack, the best friend and running partner a man could wish for

Acknowledgements

Many people have been mentioned in my memoir and credited with helping me along the way in either my running journey or helping out parents of a Type 1 Diabetic daughter, or both, and I wanted to take this opportunity to thank you again for their invaluable help, advice and encouragement. If you are not mentioned by name in the book, then please accept this as my heartfelt thanks.

Without Dr Mike " Mad Dog" Schreiber, I would not have been able to make this journey. He started as my online trainer and slave driver, and ended as a friend. Shortly after the book ends, Mike passed away, ironically on the last day of a week long ultramarathon I was participating in. You continue to be missed, Mike. I couldn't have done it without you.

Bruno, aka Victoria, at I'm Your Girl. Thanks for all your help and advice whilst penning my memoir. You helped me with constructive criticism and red ink when I needed it; you were there when struggling with structure; you provided a shoulder to cry on when I "hit the wall". I couldn't have written it without you.

And finally to my long suffering family. For the hours I spent training. Meeting me for breakfast/lunch/dinner when you drove and I ran. Following me round the mountains with cold spray, Vaseline, bandages and a hug. Standing in a puddle in the pouring rain at the barriers to cheer as I shuffled over yet another finish line. Just thanks.

Contents

4.30am 19 March 2015, Prologue

"Bip_ bip_bip_bip."
"Bip_ bip_bip_bip."
"BIP_BIP_BIP_BIP!"
"**BIPBIPBIPBIP**"

"Are you going to turn that bloody thing off or what?" Mrs R managed, simultaneously sleepy and cross.

"Oh bollocks. Sorry darling." I said, reeling from the 'tender" elbow to my solar plexus, all while fumbling with the alarm clock all. Negotiating a path in the dark over upturned bedside lamp, several books, cushions, and Jack (one of my dogs) as he performed a lazy stretch which seemed to make him three times his size, I exited from the bedroom as quickly as I could.

Half asleep, I double knotted my running shoes, and with Jack nipping at my heels, exited the house for my midweek long run. Jack and I had 21 kilometres / 13 miles of hills sprints scheduled. As we left the house, the cold and moist early morning air was better than any coffee, dusting off the cobwebs and preparing me for a new day.

I am not even sure what I am training for, a marathon in a few weeks? An Ironman triathlon a few weeks after that? An ultra or two in the more distant future? I look at one race as good training for the next; the most important thing to just keep moving forwards.

There is never any doubt about me getting up to train no matter what I have done the previous evening, how much or little I have slept. The mere act of lacing my trainers has come to define me as much as being a son, a husband or a father. I am a runner.

Of course, the upcoming race was something to train for, a reason to get up in the morning, but I run for my health and my sanity. And for the love of it.

19 June 2014, Am I Lost?

"Are you lost?"

One of the two girls slurred as they giggled past me, then half-walked half-fell across the bridge. In their early twenties, these girls were on their way home from a night spent in one of the few bars in the small town of Sospel, nestled in a deep valley cut into the Alpes Maritimes mountain range. The town was sliced in two by the river, and I had stopped next to the only bridge to fill up my backpack's bladder with water from the town fountain, and to put on some more layers as protection against the chilling humidity.

I smiled at the absurdity of it.

A middle aged man dressed in brightly coloured manmade fibres, carrying a back pack in the middle of the night in a town which had never succeeded in becoming the tourist destination it aspired to. While I may have looked lost, I knew exactly where I was and where I was going. I had arrived on a footpath, as both of the town's churches were chiming twelve, having summited the first of three mountains, or "Cols" in local parlance. I had another two mountains to climb and descend before I reached the Italian ski resort of Limone, some 70km away.

I had left my adoptive home, Monaco, four hours previously, accompanied by a minor fanfare from my wife and kids. A few of my running buddies had joined me as we trotted slowly out of Monaco and along the coastal footpath to Menton, before heading inland. Early season tourists looked over their sweating glasses of lager at us with faint smirks as we passed numerous sidewalk cafes, before reaching the industrial estate littered with broken glass and graffiti that marked the edge of the town. There my companions had called it a night, heading home for takeaway and beers, pleased with their 11km jog.

As the sun went down and the terrain went up, my adventure was just beginning.

Proceeding solo, I had embarked on an unofficial, overnight, mountainous, unsupported and unmarked 105km ultra marathon. My plan was to arrive in Limone with enough time to pin my number on, and take the start line for the Cro Magnon – a further 135km organised extreme mountain trail race which headed across the Alpes Maritimes back to the coast and the finish line on the beach just outside Monaco.

The Cro Magnon was my local ultramarathon, and I had run its baby brother, the Neander Trail, back in 2009 as my first trail ultra – a mere 50km. Having graduated to the full 114km Cro in 2010, and a host of others in the interim, I had always intended to run the re-routed and re-launched Cro Magnon in 2014.

The race had been born of one man's determination to join the twin towns of Limone, a ski resort in Italy and Cap D'Ail, a beach resort in France, which lay a few hundred metres from my adopted home. The trail traced the spice route and started at an altitude of 1000m/3000 ft, trekked over the mountains, before descending to Cap D'Ail and sea level on the French Mediterranean coast.

The towns, and the ancient trail that linked them, were steeped in history. Once upon a time traders made the journey carrying their precious cargo of spices, at the time more expensive than gold, from the East down to the coast before being shipped to other trading posts on the Med. In more recent times, cave paintings had been discovered giving birth to the race's name "Cro Magnon".

Additionally, since the route traced the border between France and Italy, it was some of the most heavily contested land in the world in the nineteenth and twentieth centuries. Second World War forts, First World War bunkers, and even earlier military installations and discarded heavy weaponry were strewn along the route. The debris is testament to the inhospitable terrain, and also adds to the sense of going somewhere few had ever been. Not to mention the added potential hazards of tripping over a half buried cannon.

Not only was the Cro Magnon a 114km / 71 mile journey from the snow to the sea, but it was also a journey through history, through time and change, and one I came to feel represented the journey I had made over the previous decade.

For the 2014 Cro Magnon, a new route had to be mapped, as one of the National Parks closed its doors to organised mass participation events, and I was drafted as an English speaking "Ambassador" for the re-launch, trying to raise awareness for the race amongst English speakers. As an Ambassador, I felt I should lead by example and immediately secured a place to run the new 130km / 81 mile route.

Already reasonably fit (having run a marathon the previous November), I began to ratchet up the training and to start fine tuning what equipment I would need to take with me for a semi self-sufficient 130km run over the mountains. Road marathons and other races tend to be like a rolling buffet with no transport provided – every couple of kilometres there are sugars, gels, chocolate, Coke – a veritable smorgasbord of short term energy hits. At the Helsinki marathon, I had been offered herring and pickles, which I politely declined. In the mountains, of course, the options were limited and even getting water to the competitors could be tough (some races rely on mules to get enough water to the competitors). As a result, the Cro Magnon had a hefty mandatory kit list of fluids, food, extra layers in case of the (highly likely) event of inclement weather, rudimentary medical supplies, compass, whistle, maps and more. My kit would eventually end up tipping the scales around 7kg.

I lived for all of this.

I relished the hours spent perusing the appropriate websites and experimenting, including cutting off labels and vacuum-packing homemade trail mix to minimise weight. Friends tell me they experienced the same pleasure in planning their hobbies whether it be golf, tennis, or motorsport; the principles of fine tuning the kit (and the pleasure derived from it) being a common passion for enthusiasts of any discipline. Whereas a golfer might search for the perfect driver, a fisherman for the perfect fly, I would search for the perfect waterproof jacket: Gore Tex, lightweight - preferably less than 250 grams, windproof, breathable, a packable hood and sealed watertight pockets. It would also be extremely compact so as to fix to the outside of my pack or even better inside with all my other equipment.

One final piece of essential kit was a small photo of my kids to give myself a morale boost if needed at the dead of night. On occasion I had pinned this to the outside of my pack. I had often been questioned by other competitors or spectators about who was in the picture, my blue eyed blonde daughters' lack of any resemblance to their dark haired grizzled father. On one occasion I had come face to face with a mountain ram who displayed similar puzzlement at the picture, or perhaps was just protecting his flock from this panting middle aged man in Lycra. Sharing a surge of paternal knowing, or perhaps merely pitying me, he retreated, following his bleating charges, into the undergrowth at the side of the path.

Planning for a mountain race had an added frisson – one wrong decision could result in not finishing the race, or even worse should there be a freak snowstorm in the middle of the night. I was acutely aware that mountains were unforgiving). Packing was definitely something I took seriously.

Perhaps more important to me than the fine tuning of the kit was the training, both mental and physical. To misquote Yogi Berra, ultra running is "90% physical, the other half mental." I had learnt from experience that the mind gave up long before the body, and there was no other way around it than weekly long training runs, some longer than a marathon.

As a husband and father of three daughters, whilst holding down a time consuming and stressful job, it was not always easy to stick to my training schedule, and the alarm would often go off at 5am and sometimes 4am in order to fit in the training kilometres. And this, of course, is why I would often jog past revellers, rolling out of the bars and clubs in Monaco. And not without relief at leaving them behind for the relative isolation of the coastal paths; one never knows what sort of drunk they will be with a fine line between friendly cheer and aggressive jeer.

On one occasion, having just started my run, I was running along the Baisse Corniche – the picturesque coastal road that links the towns from Nice to the Italian border. It was high season, flooded with tourists, well before sunrise when I noticed a smartly dressed fellow slumped against a wall which marked the other side of the road. There was no hard shoulder or pavement due to the topography, although a couple of cars were illegally parked, and the chap in question was between the two cars, the grime from the road smeared on his chinos and blazer. I waited for a quiet spot in the already busy rush hour traffic to cross the road, and check that he was ok. It had also crossed my mind that if a bus were to hit one of the cars at 80kmh / 50mph, the car would crush or decapitate the hapless reveller. I touched him gently on the shoulder as the wind from an articulated lorry threw dust into my eyes. Getting no response, I grabbed him by the arms and shook him awake. He blearily waved me away as I gagged on the alcohol fumes on his breath, but realised the gravity of the situation as a scooter hurled past us, almost touching us with his rear view mirror as he leaned into the corner. We darted across the road, and the grateful holidaymaker lurched in the direction of his accommodation, or perhaps the opposite direction, but at least he was no longer in danger of becoming pickled roadkill.

I seemed to recall a tutor in a training seminar years before telling a room full of bleary eyed and clammy skinned graduates, of which I was one, to hope for the best but prepare for the worst. That is what I was doing in preparation for the Cro Magnon. You cannot predict every eventuality, but with enough physical and mental training, you can survive anything that is thrown in your path. That physical and mental training was, in retrospect, invaluable when dealing with a wholly unforeseen challenge that was thrown at my family and me.

23 December 2013, The Storm Cometh

Dr Smith was incredibly sympathetic, but all of our suspicions were true. Alice, my 11 year old, was Type 1 diabetic. An avalanche of medical material cascaded from his arms onto the bed. I caught sight of some injection pens and some sort of handheld computer in a sealed box. The picture on the outside was a bit like a handheld games console I had had as an adolescent, in the pre-history before mobile phones. It was all I could do to get up from the uncomfortable chair and draw the curtain around our little section on the children's ward. I felt sick. My wife was wiping her eyes, and my daughter had two white streaks that the tears were leaving down her hot red cheeks.

"Why me?" she demanded, clenching the bed sheets in her fists.

"Why not someone else? It's Christmas!"

Life would never be the same again. Not for her. Nor for any of us. Two days previous, we had finished school and work, drawing a line under a difficult year. We had battled the end of term traffic to get to the airport, park, and just made our flight amidst the threat of a storm and hurricane-force winds upon our arrival in the UK. We grabbed our luggage and hired car, and with the aid of buckets of vending machine coffee, we drove through the night the 300km from the airport to my wife's parents' house. We were feeling pretty lucky, given that the forecasted apocalyptic storm had hit the airport a few hours after. Four hours after unloading the suitcases from the car, we had driven another hour to attend the wedding of my wife's sister, and we could finally relax and unwind for a few days staying over Christmas before flying back to Monaco for New Year's Eve.

Alice had lost weight going into year end, but had grown taller as kids tend to do, and our local paediatrician thought there was nothing to worry about as Alice was undoubtedly stressed about work and end of term shows. But one tiny drop of blood onto my father in law's blood glucose monitor after the wedding and we knew there was a problem.

It just said "high".

Someone without diabetes has a blood sugar level of around 5. Someone with untreated early stage Type 2 diabetes – which my father in law had developed ten years previously, might be around the 10 level. Alice was "high" which meant north of 30. I had called a local Yorkshire GP, and was told to go straight to the children's unit at York District Hospital.

We left the other two kids behind and navigated the pre Christmas traffic (and precursor to the storm that was heading inexorably northwards). I silently prayed that it was not Diabetes and tried not to think about the other – infinitely worse – diagnoses and possibilities, as I tried to deflect the inevitable "What if's" that were being shot at me in rapid succession from the passenger seat.

Dr Smith ran through a brief explanation of Type 1 Diabetes, interjected periodically by a cavalcade of crying from the infant in the adjacent bed, who was suffering from a dangerous and prolonged bout of food poisoning.

Desperate to get back to the family for Christmas, Alice very quickly took responsibility for doing her own injections and blood glucose monitoring, which necessitated a small needle prick every time. We all tried to take on board a brief education on carb counting, necessary for calculating the amount of insulin Alice would require with every meal and snack. Within a few hours we were back at my in-laws trying to process the news, with the aid of sauvignon blanc and the internet.

All sorts of thoughts were going round my head about the diagnosis, not least of which was "What if they got it wrong?" The diagnosis was very much like a bereavement, with denial being the first of five recognisable stages that we all experienced. That first night I struggled to find the positives.

24 December 2013, Christmas Gift

I woke early to check Alice's blood sugar level, and then went for a very brief Christmas Eve jog around the country lanes, whilst the kernel of an idea was already germinating in the back of my mind.

We later loaded the suitcases back into the car, feeling the weight of our extra burden. We battled with the Christmas Eve traffic driving from rural Yorkshire, to my sister in law's in rural Northumberland. Alice was feeling very positive about her condition after her own internet investigations. She now knew why her infections were not healing without medical intervention and why she was so often exhausted during the day, and that with careful management her life may actually improve. My wife, Sally, on the other hand spent the entire three hours of the journey northwards sobbing uncontrollably, so much so that I made her drink some water lest she become dehydrated.

After Christmas, we arrived back in Monaco and immediately tried to get admitted to the medical care system. We had settled into a sort of routine with the medication given to us by Dr Smith and his team, and were anxious that we would have to start over with a different regime in the French healthcare system. The same paediatrician who had previously reassured us Alice was fine, immediately prescribed us anything we wanted and agreed we should stay on the existing programme. Alice's biggest fear was that people would assume she had Type 2 diabetes – more of a lifestyle condition than a genetic condition – and use it as a tool with which to bully her. Until we could explain the situation to her school, we kept her condition to ourselves, preferring to spend New Year's Eve as a family, marking midnight with a few sparklers in the garden, angrily swishing at the misfortunes of the previous year.

Type 1 Diabetes is very rare; only 400,000 people live with the condition in the UK, less than 1% of the population. People are predominantly diagnosed when they are children or young adults, and estimates put the numbers of children with Type 1 around 35,000[1]. The numbers are more difficult to find in France, but it is comparable or even slightly less per head of population than in the UK[2]. No one knows why it occurs; various theories have been posited, but one of the common themes is that it is genetic with some sort of trigger, be it viral or a trauma. The body attacks itself, killing off the Islet cells in the pancreas that create insulin, a hormone that is necessary for the body to absorb sugars into the cells, which they then use for energy. Regardless of the cause, one day she was fine, and the next she was diabetic and her body could not process enough sugar to fuel her.

The symptoms are not always that easy to read; children grow at different rates, hence weight loss (as the body resorts to burning fat as it cannot access the sugars) can be easily explained away as growth spurts. Kids get sick and hormones can affect sleep patterns, so ongoing infections and fatigue, again, can be dismissed as part of normal growth cycles. Other symptoms can have alternate sources; extreme thirst, for example, was attributed to a poorly ventilated classroom next to a dusty building site. In the meantime, because Alice's body was burning fat for a prolonged period, it was creating something called ketones, a by-product of the fat burning process. If the ketones in her blood had been allowed to reach dangerous

---

[1] Source for both UK statistics a UK Parliamentary Speech in 2014 by Mr George Howarth,
http://www.publications.parliament.uk/pa/cm201314/cmhansrd/cm140430/halltext/140430h0001.htm

[2] Source for both UK statistics a UK Parliamentary Speech in 2014 by Mr George Howarth,
http://www.publications.parliament.uk/pa/cm201314/cmhansrd/cm140430/halltext/140430h0001.htm

levels, they could have been toxic and created something called diabetic ketoacidosis, which can result in serious illness, coma, and eventually death.

In a sense, we were lucky over Christmas. Not only had we managed to evade the "storm of the century" as one tabloid called it, with our evasive manoeuvres around England, but we had managed to diagnose Alice's condition without reaching the worst case scenario with the associated extended stay in intensive care.

Every silver lining has a cloud: we could not get into the care system until a slot came free as Alice had not been diagnosed through the normal channels – via hospitalisation, and normally intensive care. We found out that because of the rarity of the condition, Monaco hospital no longer treated Type 1 diabetes in children, and the nearest clinic was in Nice, about half an hour's drive away (and a different country). However, we could not get into the system unless Alice checked into the paediatric ward for a minimum of a week, as it was at the critically ill or even coma stage that most children in France were diagnosed. Whether this was due to lack of awareness of the condition generally, or just the difficulty of putting together enough symptoms for a diagnosis, was difficult to say.

We waited for two months before seeing a paediatrician specialising in diabetes. We were left with the cards we had been dealt, but we desperately needed assistance in the form of education and emotional support. Our denial gave way to anger, then moved to bargaining and depression in rapid succession in our mourning of Alice's pancreas.

I tried to put aside my own feelings and put my energies into doing something constructive; I knew more than Google was providing, and began thinking of a way to make connections for Alice. Her diagnosis was not, in fact, my first encounter with Type 1 diabetes.

I had spent a lot of time with two brothers not far from where I grew up, in Kent. Their father was a farmer of apples, pigs, and arable (mainly wheat and corn) at various times, and my parents joked that Sheephurst Farm was my second home because I spent so much time there. Not only did I have some male company (I had no brothers and my father was away working a lot), but the farm was a playground with space to have adventures, and lots of toys and farm vehicles with which to have them! We had some great summers there, zipping around on bikes and later motorcycles and cars that were no longer fit for the road but could be fixed up enough to trundle up farm tracks. Ever since I can remember, Nigel (the elder of the two brothers) had to check his blood, inject insulin, and eat lots of digestive biscuits. He had been diagnosed Type 1 aged around 3 or 4, but I never really understood what that meant. I could remember when Nigel swapped his glass syringes for the handy little pen, and being touched with a twinge of jealousy over the smart leather case it came in. As I had moved abroad ten years previously, I had not seen as much of Nigel and his brother, William, but had still kept in touch enough to have a drink down the pub when I was in the UK.

On Boxing Day, two days after Alice's diagnosis, I gave him a call. Alice sat next to me, still numb and speechless from the shock, but wanting to hear what Nigel had to say. Through Nigel, I learned about Diabetes UK – they had supported him throughout his life, and even funded the research into the technology that brought about the pen injector to replace the clumsy glass syringes. They offered counselling for children and their parents, and an enormous amount of education, not to mention residential weekends for families, and summer camps for the children. As Alice and I perused the website together, and Alice signed up for the Diabetes UK kids' forum, the small seed of an idea formed in my mind and began to gradually germinate, the first shoot of green was beginning to poke through.

8 January 2014, Eureka!

"Ben, come here."

"Hang on a sec, I've just walked in the door; let me take my coat off."

It was about 7pm. I was used to being attacked the minute I walked in from work with requests to help with homework, fix things, or for demands for clothes or shoes and the like. Not to mention the dogs bouncing up and down, nipping and yapping at my feet, tripping me and each other in their desperation to be acknowledged first.

"Ben, it's urgent. Now."

I stepped over the hounds, approached the kitchen, and heard the tell tale sound of a very upset offspring in the kitchen – the machine-gun-like involuntary shallow breaths, interspersed with an occasional sob. I chucked my coat in the vague direction of the nearest chair, and shot in. Alice in her mother's arms, looking very blotchy indeed.

"The Teacher" *breath*"said had I eaten" *breath*" "too many sweets" *breath*" "in front of the whole class!" she managed to get out, staccato fashion, before the tears started to flow again.

Alice had voiced this very concern the day she was diagnosed. What if people thought she herself had been the cause of her diabetes through lifestyle? She was already worried about bullies using diabetes as particularly painful ammunition. Jokes aimed at the overweight with diabetes as the punchline had been her only source of information until her own diagnosis. Type 1 diabetes, on the other hand, is like a lightning strike, a sealed fate.

I held her. It gave us both some comfort, but also stopped me from marching out the door and finding this teacher and giving him a good shake! How could someone in a position of pastoral care like that be so bloody insensitive? Even if what he had said was true (which it wasn't), he shouldn't have said it. I was so angry all I could do was splutter half sentences. I wanted to make that teacher eat his words. And anyone else who dared to speak the same.

I needed a challenge to make people sit up and really take notice, one that was so insane and beyond the realms of comprehension, that I would spark enough interest to get the message across. Her message would be my message, educating people that Type 1 was not a disease brought on by eating too many donuts. I could hold up my daughter by educating those who would put her down.

In a sense, my journey to the Cro Magnon – and back – began right there.

Not only would I run the Cro Magnon, 130km across the mountains, I decided, but I would also run to its start. Effectively doing it twice.

I wanted to divert attention away from Alice and onto me to shoulder some of the enormous burden that had been placed on her, and help her to regain her self-confidence. I wanted to make people think twice about saying something hurtful and irresponsible, including out of ignorance, as that teacher had done that day. Every child just wants to be accepted, to be normal, to belong. Alice had to draw blood and administer insulin many times a day, which made her different. If she didn't she could have a stroke, go blind, even die. I needed to do something to help Alice accept that she *was* normal, and she could control her condition rather than let it control her. And she definitely didn't have to let it define her or stop her from doing anything that she put her mind to.

I became obsessed with success stories of sportspeople and personalities with Diabetes like Sir Steve Redgrave, and their stories of overcoming the odds and inspiring others. I wanted to make my daughter - and myself - believe that anything is possible. But with the time constraints of job and family, my options were limited.

I decided to run to the start of the Cro AND run the Cro in order to prove to my daughter – and to me, that anything was possible. I had no real idea whether I could do it, as the distance would be way beyond what I had run before in the time limit required; it also included tremendous altitude change (10000m plus), and the risks of getting injured and/or lost were massive; even a twisted ankle could be potentially life threatening. The scale of the challenge hit me when I cycled about 80km of the route I would take, including hills which were so hard that I witnessed more than one defeated cyclist trudging up on foot, head bowed.

But I was committed.

25 June 2001 Fenchurch St, City of London

"Mr Rolfe, do you do any exercise?"

"Well...yes...I walk to the station every day."

"And how far is that?"

"About 500 metres".

The pudgy Indian doctor looked at me, unsmiling, over his untidy desk, and gave a little nod, as if to say "Go on".

"...and I...er...mow the lawn once a week?"

"I see; is it a big lawn?"

"Er..." I looked at my feet, not liking where this was going.

I lived in a semi-detached house in Kent with a decent sized lawn, but it only took me about 15 minutes to mow it with a self-propelled Hayter mower.

"So let me get this straight, Mr Rolfe. You smoke..." he consulted his questionnaire "20 cigarettes a day. Your alcohol consumption is on the high side, and you have a BMI which is classed as borderline 'severely overweight'".

He was referring to my Body Mass Index. It was true, since giving up club rugby to concentrate on my career, having a one year old baby, and with my wife pregnant with number two, I had let myself go a bit. I had always had a tendency to put on weight and had had various nicknames whilst growing up such as Sausage Rolfe, Billy Bunter, Keg and more recently Cream Buns, or Bunsy. It used to bother me as an adolescent but as I grew older, my priorities had shifted more towards my ability to consume pints when out with clients, and still *compus mentis* enough at the end of the night to pick up the tab.

I looked around the scruffy little Surgery. I had been despatched by my potential employer, a large UK Financial Institution, to undergo a medical before they would consummate the attractive contract that was at stake. I was one year short of 30, and since leaving University six years previously, had worked my way up through the administrative functions to being co-chief of my own team of brokers. My lifestyle consisted of travelling at least three hours every day, on my daily commute, arriving home at 8pm and then up at 4.45am the next day to go back to work. I never left the office during daylight hours; I was a stockbroker, which meant getting to the office around 6.30am, trying to come up with trading ideas mainly for my hedge fund clients, and then broking to them through the day and hopefully executing their trades. I couldn't afford to leave my desk for more than a minute or two at a time during the day in case someone sent over an order for me to execute. Orders meant money. And at the end of the day all the orders would need processing, and only then could I leave.

On a busy day I would not leave the office until 8pm or later. I gorged on Coke, coffee, burgers, and huge sandwiches at my desk on a daily basis. On top of that, several nights a week I was expected to meet potential and existing customers, and build relationships. These nights would invariably end up in a pub or restaurant, and I would get home at 12 or 1, snatch a few hours sleep and then get up to do it all over again the next day. On weekends, if I wasn't taking customers to a sporting event, I would be too exhausted to do much of anything except hang out with my young family.

"Mr. Rolfe, you need to do something about this before it's too late. If you don't, you won't see 40."
"Understood. What would you recommend?"
"It's quite simple Mr. Rolfe." he said looking at me as if I was a particularly unruly child that had been sent to the headmaster. "Lose weight and do more exercise."

The irony of what he had said had not escaped me. The Dr. was fatter than I was.

And yet, he signed and stamped my medical certificate, and I walked out of the Medical Centre with a clean bill of health, but with his words hanging over me like a threat. I had played lots of sports growing up, and although I was never what one might consider naturally talented, I had attended practises, kept fit during the season, and made the school teams in rugby, cricket, hockey and skiing, even ending up as President of my University's rugby club. I did not really pay too much attention to nutrition, eating what I wanted when I wanted, and during the summers I had a tendency to put on weight. When I left full time education I found it increasingly tough to find the time to attend practises during the week as I was working or exhausted. This had a negative effect on my performance on the pitch, so I just gave up sport completely.

The doctor's words were ringing in my ears as I walked the short distance back to my employer, but within seconds I had forgotten him. I veritably skipped the last few hundred metres to my office in order to hand in my resignation, undoubtedly the only exercise I had done that day!

20 February 2003, Kent

Despite initially trying to implement changes to my lifestyle, my gym membership was merely used to take my two daughters to the swimming pool on rainy weekends. Even then, I wasn't doing anything other than bounce the kids up and down in the shallow end until our fingers took on the texture of prunes, and then we headed for the showers and the fast food restaurant outside.

One typical week, I had been out with a client until the last train – which was invariably late. I had had a skin-full, and once at my local station I hopped over the churchyard wall to cut through the graveyard, but the weather was terrible; it was like someone was just tipping an endless bucket of water over my head. I slipped in the rain, and arrived home at about 1.30am soaking wet and covered in mud. The alarm sounded the next day at 4.45am, I showered and got into a clean suit and got the 5.15am to work. It was still raining, and mine was the only train to make it through before horrific floods stopped public transport from running. I was the only one of my team to make it in that day, and I struggled through on three hours sleep, coffee, and adrenaline. The journey home that night took five hours. I had another four hours sleep, and got up to go to work again.

Needless to say this lifestyle was not ideal. I was 16 and a half stone (238lbs or 108kg), and at 5 foot 10 (178cm's) tall, I was on the verge of becoming morbidly obese.

I was 31 years old.

The new job had not gone entirely as planned. My team had started a few days before 9/11, and before we knew it the banking system was undergoing a huge upheaval linked to money laundering in an attempt to stifle terrorist funding. My new employers decided within a matter of weeks of me joining that they really had no interest in developing that business area at all, and after being bounced around several different departments, the team and I found ourselves on a more or less abandoned area of the trading floor isolated from everyone else, with a whole encyclopaedia worth of internal regulations preventing us from actually doing anything productive.

Something had to change. I was bored and frustrated in my job, made worse by the wasted time spent getting to and from work every day. And it didn't help that I hated myself. Little things like the rash left by my thighs rubbing together and chafing if I did actually manage to walk anywhere. Mrs R was constantly moaning at the dust left in the bathroom by the liberal dowsing of talcum powder I would put on myself to counteract these irritations – it was like a forensic team had been into the bathroom every morning dusting for finger prints, and not cleared up after themselves.

18 May 2003, Moving (on)

The day after Emily's (my eldest's) third birthday, we packed up the trusty Volvo with our most precious belongings – two daughters, two cats, toothbrushes and a couple of spare pairs of underpants, and we left England. We had rented out our house in Kent, and had taken a short term lease on a place in Nice, France, whilst I had accepted a position with no salary and no expense account to join a couple of friends who were setting up a small brokerage firm in Monaco.

The attractions were endless. Better weather, no "big firm politics", no real commute, especially after things settled down and we took a two year lease on an apartment just five minutes' walk from the office. I started to have lunch once a week with the family, and Emily had settled into the local French school. We had started to meet people, developed a social life, and on weekends loved exploring the local area and popping over to Italy to visit the colourful markets.

I was still working hard. The time difference was a benefit as I could get to the office at 7.30am instead of 6.30am, and I was even more bound to the desk as there were so few of us doing everything. I even had a cordless phone and would take it to the loo with me for fear of missing orders. I was taking intensive French lessons in order to try and integrate and converse with Emily's teachers. We kept in touch with our old life in the UK by a constant stream of friends and family coming to visit, too. A full day would often be followed by a full night of dinner and entertainment, as I would get home exhausted and the guests would be winding up after a relaxing day on the beach. One old school friend (who should probably remain nameless) of Mrs R found out we had moved from Friends Reunited (a precursor to Facebook), and after not so much as a letter or email since 1990, the "great news" was that she had a couple of weeks holiday and thought she might drop in for a night or two. Fourteen days later I dropped her off at the airport, and funnily enough we didn't hear another word from her.

9 November 2003, Where there is smoke there is fire

The oppressive heat and smoke of one of the hottest summers on record gave way to a cataclysmic autumn with heavy rain on the coast and snow close enough that we could see it from our apartment, further up the cliffs that seem to push the towns of the Cote D'Azur into the Mediterranean Sea.

With the onset of the long dismal rains of November came some awful news; my Mum, previously a near neighbour in Kent and intimately involved, doting on her grandchildren, had been diagnosed with cancer.

A routine biopsy found one of the most aggressive forms of the disease, and it had spread. She needed the most aggressive treatments if she was to have a chance to beat the disease, including chemotherapy, which precluded her from travelling. She went from seeing the kids almost daily to seeing them only infrequently to seeing them almost never, in a matter of months. It would have been impractical and expensive for us to fly over to see her every weekend, but I felt the need to show some support whilst she battled both the disease and the awful side effects of the treatment.

The kids had been fed and were settled in front of the television watching cartoons – in French. I constantly had to kick myself to make sure I wasn't dreaming; one of the clear benefits of living abroad was the ability to bring up bilingual children. Emily could already speak more French than me and she was only three and a half! Mrs R was having a deserved lie in, and I was contemplating the previous few months and everything that had happened. Even though life was rosy, I had an itch that needed to be scratched.

The long hours, good food, and big, often alcoholic, dinners coupled with a lack of exercise meant that I was, if anything, in worse shape than I had been a couple of years earlier when I was given the stark warning about my lifespan. And the cancer eating away at my Mum, thankfully caught early, was another reminder of my own mortality. I sipped at my Tetley's Tea (something I wasn't prepared to leave in the UK), and gazed out over the town, through the rain, to the sea.

Immediately below me, my eyes were attracted by some very slow moving things in brightly coloured synthetics. It looked to be some sort of herd of joggers, albeit moving very slowly and a few of them had donned clear plastic sheeting as protection against the pouring rain. A few minutes later, I discovered on the fledgling internet service (this was 2003 after all), that it was the Marathon de Monaco et des Riviera. The route ran directly below my balcony. Awesome!

On the spot, I decided to run the Monaco marathon the following year, and whilst doing so raise money for Cancer Research UK, in order to give me some motivation. The cause had become very close to my heart; the more money raised for Cancer Research would give my Mum – and others like her - more chances of beating that illness. Of course, equally motivating were the obvious health benefits for me.

I bought myself some cheap trainers, put on an old pair of rugby shorts and cotton t-shirt, and went for a run. I am a morning person, so I found it easier to run before work; there were too many excuses not to run in the evening, so the mornings were preferable.

I ran before I could talk myself out of it.

I would get up early every week day – preferably before dawn so that no one would see me, put on my old stuff, trundle out the back of the apartment building, and go uphill, as direct a route as possible away from home to avoid any prying eyes.

The first time I ran, I got about 300 metres down the road, and thought I was going to have to call an Ambulance.

After dry heaving at the side of the road for a few minutes, I waddled like a Weeble for about half an hour before returning home to gorge myself on fresh warm baguette, and locally made strawberry jam.

I decided that the challenge required a bit more finesse, so after a few intensive sessions after work investigating diet and fledgling online running programs, I committed to cut down on my carbohydrates and starchy foods like bread, pasta, and potatoes.

18 December 2003, Little by little

I ran five days a week, each day a little further than the last. Within a few weeks, I had lost 10 kilos, (22lbs) not far off two stone. The difference was remarkable – not just to my wallet, as I was having to invest in a whole new wardrobe, but to my self-esteem. Not only was I raising money for Cancer Research, which could have a direct effect on my Mum's future wellbeing, but people were coming up to me and commenting about how good I looked. Mrs R and I had decided to have a little drinks party in our apartment, and it was open invite. We were really keen to meet new people and cement some relationships that were just starting to develop with acquaintances and neighbours, and I treated myself to a new jacket to mark the occasion – a lot smaller than the old one it replaced.

"Thanks so much for coming; it's lovely to see you." "Oh you shouldn't have," I'd say, as I was presented with a bottle of wine or a box of chocolates. "Thanks for inviting us. Ben, can I just say how good you are looking? The transformation since you arrived here has been remarkable; it must really suit you living here," all said while looking me in the eye and not letting go of my hand.

"No really, you look amazing! What's your secret?" asked another guest.

I attempted to extricate myself from the piston-like handshake, mumbling something about the marathon, fund raising, and diet, all in a slightly embarrassed fashion, before having to repeat it all again with the next person through the door.

Although the attention made me uncomfortable, the boost to my self confidence was remarkable. If only I had done something earlier!

12 September 2004, My first marathon

Three days after my 32nd birthday, and a couple of months before marathon day, I had pledges for several thousand pounds for Cancer Research.

I was looking and feeling better than I had been for ten years, and I was feeling really good about myself. I was using the time I had previously wasted commuting to actually extend my life, and I loved it. People continued to comment on my physical transformation, but it was not only the weight loss. I had more energy; I was able to move about and give more time and energy to my kids. Life was good.

I was extending my training runs gradually, and had run a couple of 20 milers already. At times I had to haul myself out of bed at 5am for a run, having worked a full day and then gone straight to dinner with clients before getting home in the early hours. But the negatives were far outweighed as I could tie the pain of training back to something tangible - my health, and raising money for a cause close to my heart. I also found the unexpected benefit that a bit of exercise in the morning metabolised the food and drink ingested the previous evening.

I dwelled on the changes that I had made over the previous eighteen months as I flicked through a three year old classic car magazine in my new doctor's waiting room. An easy going Dane in his mid-40's, Dr. Ritter was my family's new GP in our adoptive home. He had had a successful practise in Denmark, but had decided to flee the gloomy winters of his homeland and followed a large number of his compatriots who had settled in the South of France. I liked him because when I had landed I could not speak a word of French, and Dr, Ritter, like many Scandinavians, spoke perfect English.

"Ben! So nice to see you again! And may I complement you on how good you are looking? Life on the Cote D'Azur really suits you. What seems to be the problem?"

"Thanks Dr Ritter, that's very kind. I wish I could say it was nice to see you! You remember I am training for the Monaco Marathon?"

"Absolutely. How is the training going?"

"Well, that's the issue. It is all going really well, but I seem to have developed a pain in my shin."

I had heard about shin splints, and I had visions of Dr Ritter telling me I couldn't run the marathon, so I had put off consulting him until the pain had become unbearable. I had growing dark patches of sweat seeping from under my arms as my nerves increased.

"I don't care what I have to do, I just want you to get me to that start line."

Ritter would understand; he was a keen cyclist and had followed my marathon training with interest. "I completely understand. I would like you to go straight to the hospital next door and I will arrange an x ray and an MRI scan on your ankle and shin, and see if we can find out what the problem is. Then we will make a decision."

I wasn't sure what to think as I returned a few hours later with the massive envelope full of pictures of my leg. It was too much to bear thinking about not starting the marathon; I had so much invested and so many funds raised. Even if I had to hop it on one foot, I was determined to get round. My Mum's treatment had ultimately been successful; she was in remission and had been given clearance to come to Monaco and watch the race.

Ritter gently explained that the sheath that houses the tendons in the front of my shin had become inflamed, which was ironically good news. The condition, often confused with shin splints, was a relief. I had visions of looking at fractured bones on the x ray negatives, (occasionally that can happen) – a stress fracture, which was extremely painful. In my case, the pain was comparable; it felt like someone was stabbing me with a red hot dagger every time I moved the ankle, but I was reassured that with a month's rest, ice, anti-inflammatory gels, and more rest, and I would be at the start line just outside the Casino in Monte Carlo.

In one sense, it was a relief. In another, a huge worry.

I had been training for almost a year, and I knew that fitness and what conditioning I had achieved would disappear in a flash, compared with how long it had taken to gain it. What if I managed to get to the start line but didn't have enough fitness to finish the race? The course itself was hilly with a huge climb from Menton up to the road that led back into Monaco, and to top it all off, because of the logistics of organising a race which went from Monaco into France and Italy, before coming back, the organisers had to implement tight time limits so that the various police forces could reopen the roads to traffic. For months I had been having a recurring nightmare where I was forced to quit by the sweeper.

Oh, the sweeper bus!

There was an actual bus with a witch's broom tied to the front that followed the runners at the slowest allowed speed. If it overtook a runner, a marshall would exit the bus, take the number and timing chip from the runner, and then encourage the exhausted and utterly dejected runner onto the bus. I was waking up in the night in a sweat with the horrors of being forced onto the sweeper bus; the humiliation and sense of letting everyone down only slowly dissipating once I realised it was a nightmare.

I became, if anything, more determined. I walked everywhere, joined a gym and cycled one legged frantically 7 days a week, to the bemused glances from other, more serious, gym members. I started going to the beach and braving the decreasing sea temperatures, splashing around one-legged, just off the beach, swimming in circles. The week before the marathon I started, gingerly, to run again. I ran 25km the Sunday before the marathon, and whilst I was slow, I was able to keep a steady pace without stopping for a rest. I hoped that that would be enough to carry me through.

Seven days later, I hobbled arthritically up the ramp into the Stade Louis II.

The Monaco cheerleading team, in matching cheerful costumes in the Monaco red and white, greeted me with chants I had neither the energy nor vocabulary to translate, but their enthusiasm was welcomed and contagious. I managed to muster a pathetic trot to circumnavigate the grassy infield, the spongy track surface a welcome relief after the brutal 4hrs 26 minutes of tarmac on my screaming legs and shins. Tears of joy and pain streamed from my eyes, matched by twin tracks of blood staining the front of my Cancer Research UK t-shirt. My nipples had rubbed raw and were freely bleeding. I had nothing left to give, having intermittently walked and jogged the last ten kilometres of the marathon. At points, it felt like old ladies with zimmer frames could have overtaken me, I was travelling so slowly. I was bursting with a mixture of pride and pain, and the atmosphere of the stadium with cheerleading friends and family encouraging the last finishers.

I collapsed into the arms of the two Mrs. R.'s – my wife and Mum – and the latter, who had been known to cry at TV Commercials, was in danger of serious dehydration. My wife, coming from Yorkshire, was less well known for her public displays of emotion, but I could see deep pride in her eyes. The kids, perhaps still too young to really understand what I had achieved, were just happy to see me.

I didn't take off my medal for days afterwards, wearing it alongside a general disbelief that I had actually completed a marathon, which meant that I continued to receive donations for Cancer Research long after the stiffness had left my legs, busting through my target of £1000[3].

---

[3] I have used www.justgiving.com as an online platform to raise money ever since my first effort which was all paper based – it takes out the hassle of chasing everyone for money and people can add Gift Aid if a UK tax payer

With this sense of achievement, though, came a new, nagging doubt.

It was like a scab that would not heal. I wanted to have another go – to break the magic milestone of 4 hours that seemed to be the holy grail of the amateur marathon runner in every running magazine and internet forum I read.

With nothing definitive on the horizon, though, I started to slip back into my old routine. It became easier to hit the snooze button and go back to sleep in the mornings rather than go for a run. My jeans started to get a little tighter, and I found myself looking forlornly at the used belt hole a notch, and then two, from the one I was used to wearing.

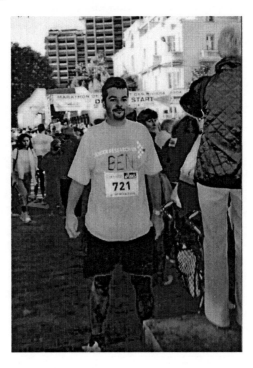

Nervous before the gun - Photo by Carolyn Rolfe

19 June 2014, Wildlife on the Col de Brouis

The sound of something heavy stepping clumsily through the undergrowth roused me from whatever zone I was in, if I was even in one, as it was about 2.30am. My heart rate quickened. I had left Sospel, and the last intermittent human habitation behind a couple of hours previously, and was trudging my way up the Col de Brouis, an almost vertical kilometre from the valley below. I was skirting several different national parks, and I no longer had reception on my mobile phone, but I knew that if I did not investigate the rustling I would regret it for a lifetime.

The worst case scenario was that it was another human, attracted by the glow of my headlamp in splendid isolation, and whoever it was, and most likely intended to empty my pockets. I parted from the flock of fireflies that had decided to accompany me for part of the climb, and headed over to the thick wood that bordered the path.

Two eyes reflected back at me like laser points, caught in the beam of my LED, and I recoiled from the smell.

It smelled distinctively gamey, so strong I could taste it. In front of me, about a metre / three feet away, was a wild boar, as shocked at my sudden appearance as I was at his. My heart rate went up several more notches when the light glinted off his tusks. I had never encountered a wild boar before, except with some strong mushrooms and a savoury red wine gravy. My only other knowledge of them was gleaned from *Asterix and Obelix* books as a child, and horror stories replayed on TV documentaries, or in the tabloids.

What the bloody hell was I thinking? I hadn't even considered the wildlife in my extensive planning of my trip. I should have brought a knife or something to make a loud noise with. Mrs. R. would never forgive me if I was gored by a wild animal and bled to death on the side of a mountain pursuing some idiotic Boys' Own adventure.

This particular fellow was more interested in his stomach than he was in me, and, with surprising speed, he scuttled a couple of metres in the opposite direction, resuming his grunting and sniffing at the base of a tree. From the slope below, I could hear some more grunting and snapping twigs, and after an aborted photo attempt (which merely seemed to capture the beast's disembodied, laser-like eyes), I jogged back up to the path.

It was important for me to stop and take in the scenery and wildlife as I went. I was on a deadline, to get to Limone and register for the Cro Magnon, eat and perhaps grab a few hours of sleep. But I knew that the key to completing the challenge was pacing. Stopping to take the odd photo or investigate a rustling in the bushes was helping to slow me down, and ironically, would actually speed me up. The story of the tortoise and the hare was real.

That pig – and my new buddies the fireflies - weren't the first examples of wildlife I had encountered that evening. As night had fallen, a lot of animals had come out to play. I had a lot of time on my hands to think, and I had plumbed the depths of my knowledge gleaned from GSCE biology and BBC nature programmes. As a result, I felt I was getting quite good at deciding which animal was which just by the spacing of their eyes and the colour of the lasers firing back at me when my headlamp reflected on the rear of their retinas.

Cats were pretty easy to identify having small heads, and forward facing eyes tinted a yellowy green. I could see where the name "Cats' Eyes" had come from for the reflectors in the middle of British roads. When I saw three pairs of bright green lasers firing at me at the side of the road on the top of the Col de Castillon, I was more intrigued. Slightly larger than cats, they could have been small dogs, but when I got close enough to see their bodies, I realised I had encountered a group of young badgers, play-wrestling. A smile played on my lips as they

34

decided I wasn't a threat, and they carried on their adolescent hi-jinks.

I had already seen much more wildlife that night than I had in my participation in more than ten ultra marathons. I would normally have been behind the (often salaried and sponsored) front runners in any organised race, so any wildlife that was out would normally have been scared away by the repeated thundering of a herd of humans on the trails.

But this time, I was in the LEAD.

I continued my climb up the Col de Brouis, marvelling at the amount of stars in the sky as I left the light pollution of humans far behind me. The Auberge at the top of the Col was the only man made structure for miles but it was almost 900 metres above sea level, about 2500 feet or so. The difference in temperature to the coast, and even Sospel, was startling. I was billowing increasingly large clouds of steam with every breath and was glad I had put on all my spare layers back in the valley. The last thing I needed was the clamminess next to my skin causing a chill in the damp mountain night. But the humidity and cold was having an unexpected, and unpleasant, side effect. The soles of my feet felt hot, possibly blistering.

I had used the same type of socks to run in over the last ten years for everything; the cheap and cheerful Run500s from Decathlon, and was very comfortable in them, so much so that I even wore them with a suit to work (especially helpful when I pounded the pavements between offices on marketing trips). They had become like a second skin. A few months before the Cro Magnon they had changed the design and they were a little thinner. I had never suffered from bad blisters in my entire running career; even when crossing the Sahara, I had developed only three. The only reason I could think of was that the humidity and cold had shrunk my feet slightly, and coupled with the thinner socks my feet were floating around inside my shoes, creating hot spots which would lead to blisters.

I was so wrapped up in my ailments that I lost the path, even though I could see the lights of the Auberge up above me. Using my hands to cling to any available foliage, I scrambled the last few metres up a near vertical bank, getting drenched in the process from the dew that had soaked into the long grass. I sat down at a picnic table (the Auberge had long ago closed for the night) and debated my options. I had no spare socks, no blister kit, it was 3am, and I was miles from any civilisation. My mobile phone reception was patchy at best, and the chances of me getting anyone out of bed, driving an hour or so with a spare pair of socks up a mountain were somewhere between slim and none. I couldn't believe I had been so stupid; I thought I had prepared for everything, but I had become so used to running with very few blister problems that that my carefully prepared kit was lacking.

I took my shoes and socks off to inspect the damage and dry my feet. I breathed a small sigh of relief when I could see no real signs of damage. They felt a lot worse than they looked, but I was not sure whether that was a good thing or not. I dried them, paying extra attention to between the toes, with a spare Buff, and put my now soaking and cold socks and shoes back on.

I took a suck on my fluids, taking note that I did not really have too much of that left either, and ruminated with some homemade trail mix. I had seen a standpipe a few hundred metres down the track, for livestock, and could fill up my bladder there. I was not sure how drinkable the water was though, compared to the "Eau potable" signs in many of the villages in the area. Breil was the next town along, and I knew there were drinking water options there. It was all downhill from the Col which meant expending less energy, not getting as hot, needing less fluids, and maybe not dehydrating. I decided to risk it, and without further ado, jogged over the edge of the Col into the Roya valley.

The descent began with a series of switchbacks to counter the steep terrain, and there was no real path so I stuck to the main road, traffic not being an issue at that time of night. I was wakened from a "daydream" by the appearance of two pinpricks of light about 200 metres / 500 feet away from me. This time the eyes were different. They were spaced further apart than I had seen before, but seemed to be forward facing, ruling out a deer or small horse. I knew from wildlife documentaries that carnivores had forward facing eyes to gauge the distance when pouncing on prey, whereas herbivores', such as horses and cows, eyes sit on the side of their heads in order to increase their field of vision whilst grazing to avoid being eaten by a predator. At night it was very common to see only one eye from a deer or even sheep. Perhaps that was where the expression "keep an eye open" had come from?

The spacing and very vague outline of the animal ruled out it being a dog, as it was just too big. Besides what would a dog be doing at the top of a mountain with no human habitation other than the Auberge which was several kilometres behind me? My heart rate increased as I cycled through the possibilities like the images on a slot machine, and as the cylinders came to a halt in my mind, the image of a large, grey, slavering wolf was the only one I was left with. I decided not to investigate further, and increased my strides to match my pulse. I rounded the next switchback, and tearing my headlamp away from whatever was watching me to highlight my route, I caught a glimpse of another one directly in front. I turned around to make sure they weren't one and the same, and my fast jog turned into a sprint! Whatever it was, there were two, one in front and one behind. I hoped that the lamp would provide some sort of deterrent to whatever they were, and the fact I was sticking to a route which should not trouble them, provided they remained stationary, meant I would soon leave them both behind.

I breathed a sigh of relief when, a short time later, I could see the orange glow leeching into the sky from the town of Breil sur Roya. I was panting and I slowed for fear of blowing up and becoming the hare in the old fable. The

37

danger – whether real or imagined – was sufficiently behind me. Whether they were wolves, mountain cats, or the large guard dogs that shepherds in the Italian/French mountains left to guard their herds, a close encounter with any would not have been pleasant, and I did not regret not stopping to take a selfie with them.

13 November 2005, Man Down

"Go...on....without...me!" David shouted at me, in between dry heaves at the side of the road.

"C'mon David, you can do it. It's not far now, only another 8km, 5 miles. How many 5 milers have you done in training? Come on."

"Leave me. Oh God, I'm going to die!" David exclaimed as his whole body shook with another violent retch.

"I'm not leaving you now. We've gone this far together. We're going to finish together. Come ON!" I commanded.

David pulled himself together as much as he could, and started slowly shuffling over the border from France to Monaco. Thankfully, after a few metres we hit the downhill next to the Country Club, the sun glinting off the waves, looking like sparkling diamonds on the sea below us. I certainly didn't feel too sparkly, apart from the salt crystals that had appeared from the dried sweat on my t-shirt, and David looked even worse.

It was a brutally hot day, and as I looked at my watch I realised we weren't going to break the four hour barrier no matter what we did. I adjusted my goals and decided to stick with David to the bitter end. There were more important things in life than personal time goals.

22 February 2005, Spider In A Jar

"Oh my God, I'm going to die."

My legs went to jelly, and I grabbed the kitchen counter, passing the phone to my wife without even cutting the connection.

"What? What's happened?"

"They want me back in tomorrow."

"What for?" The colour drained from her face.

"She wouldn't say. Just that I have to go back to the skin specialist tomorrow, to chat with the doctor."

It was a cloudless afternoon in February, so typical of the Cote D'Azur, (and part of the reason we had moved to the South of France) the exact opposite to the incoherent jumble that occupied my brain. The week before we had taken our first holiday since relocating, a week's skiing in the Alps, and I finally had a chance to tell Mrs. R. about a freckle that had been bothering me on my upper arm. It was unbelievably itchy, like a mosquito bite that wouldn't go away. With impressive speed (unlike my previous marathon attempt), the GP had referred me to a dermatologist, and after initially dismissing it as nothing but a freckle, he removed it, inserting a stitch to stop the bleeding. I was already feeling better, until the phone call.

After a sleepless night spent worrying and trying to think about something else – anything else - I went back to the dermatologist with Mrs. R. providing moral support. The doctor, brusque and dismissive, explained briefly that the biopsy had shown some pre-cancerous cells. Within a few minutes I was back in his chair looking at a large chunk of my arm that sat in a jar of clear liquid on his desk, with the stitch he had inserted into it the previous day, looking like a dead spider. He had excised a 4cm (1.5 inch) strip of flesh about 2.5cm (1 inch) across and had gone down to the muscle. I would have to have quarterly checkups for the next few years, but with any luck the bad stuff had not spread.

A couple of weeks after I had been sent home with a big hole in my arm, I returned to have my stitches out, and pick up the results of the second surgery. I was given the all clear. They had managed to get all the offending cells, and it had not spread anywhere else. I was very fortunate to have picked up on the abnormality at a very early point in its development, and absolutely did the right thing in having it removed when I did.

Life went on.

But it reinforced my desire to stay on my healthier path and also to "Carpe Diem".

13 November 2005, Staying The Course

David and I ran (in our minds, I was sure that the well-wishers watching would have called it shuffling, waddling, anything other than running), along the seafront in Monaco, the superyachts gently bumping each other on our left, and the mixture of art deco and seventies high rise on our right.

It was just a question of gritting our teeth and getting through it.

Despite the fact that I was much happier than David–he had since lost the power of speech and was wincing with every step – the simple fact of being on my feet in constant motion for four hours meant that every nerve ending was screaming at me to stop. At the nearest point of the race to my apartment, Mrs R and the kids were there to cheer us on. The rest of the crowds had long since dissipated, as the field had spread out to such an extent that David and I were running on our own. Their faces were an instant pain killer. I was able to focus on something positive. When I got up that morning I was not even sure I was going to make the start line, let alone the finish line, as Mrs R was 9 months pregnant.

After my brief encounter with the dismissive dermatologist, even though I had planned to run the marathon, Mrs R and I had decided to *Carpe Diem* and try for baby number 3. Secretly I hoped for a boy, but, like every parent, would be happy with a healthy baby, whichever flavour. Mrs R fell pregnant almost immediately and the due date fell on marathon day. Despite the precarious timing of the race and the risk that I would not be able to run it, neither Mrs. R. nor I felt at all anxious. There was a serenity about the impending chaos that we were not only familiar with, but looking forward to. It was like the proverbial calm before the storm. As a result, I had had no pre-race nerves; the year had been momentous on multiple counts, and as the race approached I had been remarkably relaxed.

It was, of course, a relief that she did not appear to have gone into labour since the race began, and I encouraged David as we arthritically shuffled towards the Stade. David's family were there to cheer us on as we crossed the finish line, and with eyes brimming over, David and I embraced.

We had crossed the line in around 4 hours 10 minutes. I was amazed, because the initial euphoria I had felt at crossing the line the first time the previous year was the same. I was so glad I had finished, mainly just to give my aching body a break, but all the work, training and dedication, and the relief and joy brought tears to my eyes. My finisher's photos should be legendary because they were all so awful. I knew then that I was hooked. I signed up right then for the 2006 Monaco Marathon.

I still hadn't cracked the magic four hours, but that could wait. We shared a hot Thai curry that night, David and me and our respective other halves, and the spices seemed to do the trick; Mrs R gave birth to our third daughter Isabelle (Izzy) at home a couple of days later.

19 June 2014, This Little Piggy

I had been trying to ignore the pain in the soles of my feet. I had put Breil between myself and the "wolves" and was sticking to the main road, inexorably uphill, towards Limone. I had driven the road many times, and cycled up it once on pre-race reconnaissance, and I knew it reasonably well. The traffic was restricted to massive juggernauts, sending shockwaves over me when they overtook, as they negotiated the tight bends at death defying speeds. Wherever possible I took paths at the side of the road, but short of heading up into the wilderness, I had to stick to the valley floor. On one such excursion, I rounded a bend and disturbed a huge wild boar with five or six piglets, snuffling alongside the path. I was close enough to touch her, and having seen David Attenborough's warnings in numerous documentaries about wild animals protecting their young, I jumped up and sideways simultaneously. Before I had even landed, my legs were already pumping. I landed slightly off balance, exacerbated by the rucksack, and with a worrying twinge in my side, I sprinted at speeds that probably would not have worried Usain Bolt but felt quick to me.

As I headed uphill and away from the sow, I had managed to land behind two piglets which were squealing and sprinting as fast as their laughably out of proportion legs could carry them. The path was, as usual, wooded and overgrown on both sides and cut into the soil from hundreds of years of walkers and hikers. It was more like a narrow channel than a path, and there was nowhere to go. I had an angry mother and a few piglets behind me, and two terrified piglets in front of me.

Panicked squeals in front, angry grunting behind. I carried on sprinting. At least my mind had been taken off my burning feet.

After a moment, the baby pigs tired, and flopped into the undergrowth impervious to thorns, allowing me to overtake. I could still hear grunting behind me but it faded as I put distance between the babies and me. Once again I carried on at a fast clip until I judged it safe, then slowed to a walk to recuperate.

Thursday 19 June 2014, Middle Aged Men In Man Made Fibres

Over the years, as I became more involved in endurance running, I made many new friends. Some I hadn't even met in person; ah the wonders of social media. During my training I had been contacted by a lawyer from Austria who regularly holidayed in Menton. Intrigued by my fund raising and more so by my impending challenge, he had invited me to accompany him for a short run in Menton. I timed meeting him with a midweek long run, ran to Menton, met him at the far side of the beach promenade, and we jogged back towards Monaco together.

It was great fun for me, breaking up the monotony of many lonely miles, especially considering it was before dawn on a Wednesday, and I hope great fun for Michael, to meet and run with someone new whilst away from home and friends.

I had similarly been contacted by a near neighbour, a transplanted Finn living just outside Monaco, who had entered one of the Ultra Trail of Mont Blanc support races. He was regularly travelling to Limone for mountain trail training, and had offered to support me in my pre-Cro challenge. I had never met him before, but texted him from Breil, and we arranged to meet about 4.30am a little further up the valley.

Not long after the pig incident, it was this man Markus who pulled up in his van to dispense Coke and moral support. I rested my weary body on the tailgate of his van, and sipped from the cup that I clipped to my back pack. I gave Markus a very brief précis of my adventures and, adhering to the ultra-mantra, "Beware the chair", thanked him and went on my way.

I felt like a new man. My feet no longer hurt, my body didn't ache, and I wasn't bone weary. It never failed to amaze me that a few words and a friendly face, not to mention a cup of Coke, was as good as a bath, three hearty courses, and a good night's sleep. Of course, the effects of the former were not as long lasting as those of the latter, but for a time I felt like a new middle aged man in manmade fibres.

Friday 10 November 2006, If at first you don't succeed

David and I were each munching on a generously proportioned bowl of pasta, outside a touristy cafe in Monaco. We both had an Asics plastic carrier bag next to us, filled to the brim with all the free marathon goodies, as well as our race numbers. It was the tenth anniversary of the Marathon de Monaco et des Riviera, and to mark the occasion the organisers had pulled out all the stops. It was our first free Technical T-shirt we had received – a natty black and gold offering to mark the important anniversary.

The registration process was now second nature to me, having turned up to the "Expo" (a cross between a retail outlet dedicated to sports and sporting events, and the place where athletes signed in and picked up their race numbers) with my medical certificate stating I was fit to run. For insurance purposes in France, all participants have to have a medical certificate after varying degrees of examination from a doctor; my doctor, after the initial examination, merely asked me if I had trained and stamped a template for me, for a nice fee, naturally. I swapped my medical certificate for a number, or *dossard* in French, and then went to collect the free stuff! My bib had been drawn in the raffle, and I had won a set of wine glasses. I was feeling lucky. Whilst there was an array of stalls selling everything you could ever want or need to enable you to do sport, David and I bypassed these heading straight to lunch.

I had trained well and had also entered every single race I could in the lead up, including the Great North Run – the World's Biggest Half Marathon - held in Newcastle every year. Mrs R had caught the bug; her sister lived in Newcastle, and we had combined a long weekend with her relatives, leaving the kids with her nephews for a couple of hours, and ran the race together. The atmosphere was amazing: the streets were lined the whole way, and little kids alternately sprayed the runners with hose pipes, or offered jelly babies from their posts on the road in front of their houses.

I had decided to raise money for Cancer Research UK again, combining the half marathon in late September with the full marathon about six weeks later. I thought that as this was my third marathon, people would be more inclined to donate if I extended the challenge; 63km / 39 miles sounded much more impressive than a *mere* marathon. I was also hell bent on beating the four hour mark.

There wasn't much to discuss over lunch. David and I had done most of the long training miles together, finding the company a very effective distraction from aching muscles and joints. All that was left was to get a decent night's sleep, remember to double tie our shoe laces, and to avail ourselves of the facilities before the start of the race.

Sunday 12 November 2006, Scaling "The Wall"

David and I were jumping up and down in front of the Casino, wrapping our arms back and forth around our bodies to keep warm. It was 8am, and whilst not raining, there was a little humidity and it was chilly. We were at the back of the pack - albeit a very small pack - and we were waiting patiently for the start, laughing and joking nervously.

I was feeling confident, having dipped below 80kg / 176 lbs for the first time, although it had been a huge struggle. I had spent most of my adult life a lot larger, and therefore my body was always metabolising what I put into it to try and go back to the "stasis" level, a bit like a wet sponge that regained its shape once pressure was no longer applied. As a result I had made a real effort to change my ways: educating myself about the food groups, and cutting out bread, pasta, and rice. I had found that I needed motivation to help me to try and keep the weight off, as it was far too easy to revert to my old ways. The marathon, and my four hour target, became my motivation.

From our vantage point at the back of the pack, David and I could see Prince Albert of Monaco, and Paula Radcliffe the British and World Record holding marathon runner, take the balcony above Barclays Bank overlooking the Casino. I can neither confirm nor deny that I "watered" a tree in Casino Gardens (at any other time an arrest-worthy offence) along with about 100 other runners, as the excitement and over-hydration got to me. Then Paula fired the starting pistol, and the noise of running shoes shuffling on tarmac and the tinny hissing of iPods became deafening. David and I whooped and hollered our excitement at Paula when we trotted past, and then it was time to concentrate on the job at hand.

My research before this race had delved into race strategy, as a new addition to formulating a proper training plan. All the forums and blogs mention something called "The Wall", the point at which it becomes virtually impossible for the runner to continue due to exhaustion. I had reached "The Wall" back in 2004, and watched David hit it, hard, in 2005. I thought that if I were to successfully break four hours, I needed to be in condition good enough to comfortably run the race. What I did not realise at the time was that race strategy also makes up a massive part of a marathon – or any – race. I had consciously learnt, however, that marathons should be started slowly – "at conversational pace" was an oft used phrase. For the first few kilometres, therefore, I was happy to shoot the breeze with David.

The route was unchanged from previous years, heading along the main road just over the border into France, veering off down the steep hill past the Monte Carlo Country Club (which is, confusingly, in France), looping back into Monaco and then along the beach front. After 3km / 2 miles, or so, we headed up a small ramp into a tunnel which was, on any other day, the main traffic artery through Monaco, and then up the same Country Club Hill to the Baisse Corniche in the direction of Italy. After so many short, energy sapping hills, the field was thinning out substantially and David and I were able to run freely, albeit still chatting.

Occasionally we would meet someone else and encourage them along, most of the runners being tourists combining their love of marathons with a short holiday. One was wearing a 100 marathon club t-shirt - from the UK, and we took the opportunity to ask for a few tips. Stunned, we watched as he rolled a cigarette from a pouch he had tucked into his shorts, and proceeded to smoke it whilst he ran. He counselled us to take it easy for as long as possible, and to enjoy the distractions.

The course had become very familiar – not just because of my prior participation but also because most, if not all, my training had been done covering the same piece of tarmac. We cheered the mainly Kenyan front runners as we ran along the sea front in Menton – they were coming the other way already two thirds into their race. The Italian border no longer required passports, so the old passport control kiosks stood quietly eroding at this now party zone of bands. A kindly elderly gent dressed entirely in tweeds offering runners and passers-by disposable cups filled to the brim with red wine. I politely declined.

Turning round at the familiar spray painted curved line on the road, just shy of Latte, we headed back up the hill on the home lap. The whole way we had been leapfrogged by an enthusiastic fellow runner stopping to take selfies of himself against various backdrops. He stopped to catch the sun glinting over his shoulder, checking the screen on his digital camera to see whether the picture would suffice, and on the other side of the road – a little behind us, still on his out lap - was a man with what looked like a curved metal blade replacing one of his legs. Inspired, we jogged on.

David stopped to stretch, and dropped back just before crossing the border from Italy back into France. His training had not been as steady as mine and he had suffered from a virus which had curtailed his training about a month before the race. As agreed, I would carry on with my goal to break four hours. I wished him luck over my shoulder, and trotted on, muscles aching but not yet in crisis.

But as I passed Menton's Port Garavan for the second time, my muscles were starting to ache. Without warning, a man in front of me stopped, and carrying the momentum of almost 30km / 18.5 miles in my body, I struggled to avoid bashing into his back and muttered expletives under my breath. As I less than deftly sidestepped him, I realised he was pushing a jogging buggy complete with a real live baby, and he was starting to change his baby's nappy. Only a few minutes later and he passed me by, baby happily gurgling and pointing at nothing. He still had to push the heavy baby and buggy combination up "Hernia Hill" – a name David and I had given it in training because we were barely able to muster more than a steady walk up it. I never saw "Super Dad" again.

As I crested the last real hill in Cap Martin, still around 8 kilometres / 5 miles from the finish, I was trying to calculate what pace I needed to run in order to break four hours, using only my analogue watch. Ordinarily, this would not have caused me many issues, mental arithmetic being an innate part of my job, but 34km / 21 miles into a marathon and I struggled to form any sort of coherent thought process. There were pockets of spectators, long since cheered out, but I did my best to get some sort of encouragement from them as I went past, gesticulating with my hands. Any smile or wave was a morale booster, and I needed all the help I could get. I was having to work really hard to keep moving and push all the negativity to the back of my mind; a little voice was whispering that it was ok to stop and rest for a while; maybe walk a few metres or a kilometre; the four hour mark was just a number. Getting a rise from a bystander was like a shot of adrenaline: a pain killer and energy booster rolled into one wave or cheer. More importantly it enabled me to ignore the "devil-voice" in my head.

Mrs R had agreed to come to a local landmark -the Meridien Hotel, not far from our apartment - and be there to cheer me on and give me a boost for the final few kilometres. We had calculated a likely time when I would be passing, but when I reached the Meridien, she wasn't there. I had a momentary lapse of morale and motivation; I stumbled, then I looked at my watch, and in a rare moment of clarity and comprehension, I realised that I had reached the Meridien ahead of schedule.

I tried to focus on keeping my momentum and achieving my goal, mainly because it would entail some rest. But I was distracted by the thought that Mrs R and the kids must have arrived at the Meridien after I had passed it, were waiting for me, getting increasingly annoyed. As I emerged from the tunnel under the Rocher, the Stadium dominated the skyline. I caught sight of David's family. I ran past, shouting that David was ok, but could someone call Mrs. R. and let her know I was almost done.

From there it was a short, painful climb up the ramp into the stadium, past the enthusiastic cheerleaders complete with red and white pompoms, and then a lap of the track, blissfully padded after the miles and miles of unforgiving tarmac and pavement.

I crossed the line in 3 hours and 54 minutes.

One of the red-tracksuited volunteers approached me with a look of pride and pleasure as she recognised my achievement. She peeled off one of the medals, getting ready to drape it round my neck, but her expression turned to concern when she saw my face. Like one of Pavlov's dogs, the finish line had the same effect as previously; my eyes had filled with tears. Coupled with total exhaustion, my euphoria and emotion were making it hard to breathe.

It was like an asthma attack. My body started to convulse in efforts to breathe, but my airway was constricted, preventing much needed oxygen. I was grabbed on both sides by fleece clad marshals and dragged to the medical tent, a few metres away.

As I crossed the threshold of the medical tent I was guided by a white coated medic and shoved into a metal folding chair. Within a few seconds I managed to control my emotions and my airways opened up. I was given a quick once over by the medic before being allowed to go and retrieve my medal, and head home, all the while worried about Mrs R waiting for me. Every step hurt, but the pride and sense of achievement acted like an anaesthetic as I hobbled through the maze of tunnels in the stadium to make for the exit.

The exertion had taken everything out of my body, and once outside, I was freezing to the point of having to borrow some money from David's wife to buy myself an additional t-shirt. She had thankfully called Mrs. R., who was making her way back home again with the three kids, and I was able to wait and cheer David in to the finish. He shuffled past a few minutes later, sweating and broken. For the second year running, he had failed to break four hours and was not only knackered but bitterly disappointed.

For my part, I revelled in my achievement for a few days. But as time went on, I felt like there was a hole in my life; for three years I had been chasing a dream, and now I had reached it. Now there was, in its place, a growing sense of unease.

Thursday 19 June 2014, Solo But Not Alone

The sky was slowly turning milky white. The sun was coming up, but dawn in Alpine valleys was a slow affair, as the mountains raised the horizon that much higher. I was jogging slowly into Tende, my feet killing me, and not really warming up despite the presence of the sun. I sat down outside a cafe, not yet open for business, but the presence of three wizened old mountain men outside suggested it would not be too long. I had promised myself a coffee and croissant to cheer myself up once I reached Tende, but that could wait. The morale boost from Markus' pit stop had long since passed, but I tried to dwell on the positives. Mrs R had woken up and had managed to pass some fresh socks and blister kit to another friend, Martin, who had promised to come up and support my insane solo challenge.

In the meantime, I dug out the number of Elio Bottero, one of the Cro organisers and a well-known Limone native. He had managed to secure me a pass to run through the tunnel – hewn from the rock by Napoleon prior to his invasion of Italy – that marked the border between France and Italy. There was no other way to make the crossing, unless I climbed the Col de Tende, which would effectively add another half marathon, not to mention the extra 1000m / half a mile of altitude, to my journey. I had asked the border police on the French side whether I could run through the tunnel, but they had said no. In preparation for my challenge, I mentally prepared myself to go over the Col.

Whilst at work, the day of my departure, Pietro, the head of the Cro committee, called me and said that the Col was under so much snow that the summit was impassable. The route for the Cro itself had been subject to a number of changes as a result, and competitors would be going on a more circuitous path in the initial stages to avoid the higher ground. My idea was to run to the start of the race, but not necessarily run the course in reverse. I was taking a slightly more direct route, some of it on the roads. I was after all on an unsupported night time traverse of the mountains. There were some risks I wasn't comfortable taking, and getting lost in a snowstorm up a mountain with no support was not one of them. For obvious reasons I was trying to get to Limone in the most direct way possible.

The good news was that Elio had pulled some strings with the Italian side of the border, and if he drove behind me they would let me run through. I had driven through the tunnel many times when heading to Limone for a day's skiing. The tunnel itself was narrow – a throw-back to a life before cars - and there were frequent crashes as the mad dash to the slopes on a Friday or home on a Sunday became more important to some than safety. When the tunnel was closed, the only other route available to cars was via Cuneo – a horseshoe of a journey which took an extra four hours or so. The tunnel had recently become single file, with a lengthy wait for the traffic lights to change, and queues could build up.

I was scheduled to call Elio from Tende so that he could leave Limone in plenty of time to drive through the tunnel from Italy to France, and then drive behind me as I ran the 3km / 2 mile under the mountain from France into Italy. When his sleepy and heavily accented voice answered the phone, it was merely to impart more bad news. The border police had conferred with head office, since my conversation with Pietro about 14 hours previously, and they had completely overturned the decision to allow me to cross through on foot. I was on my own again as my inner debate raged:

"Come on Ben. The sooner you crack on, the better."

"Oh pleeeease! Just five more minutes. The cafe will be open then. I could get a croissant and a cafe au lait. I'll warm up and then I'll leave. I mean, what's another half an hour in the grand scheme of things?"

"No! You have to leave! NOW!"

"Whyyyyy? There's no point. I can't go over the Col and I can't go through the tunnel. How am I going to get to Limone? Hitch a lift? There's no traffic anyway. It'll pick up in an hour or two...perhaps I could even get an hour's sleep..."

It would have been easy to let my head go down and sit and wait for the cafe to open, in the vain hope of cheering myself up with some caffeine and junk food. But I suspected that this would probably have the opposite effect. I would stiffen in the cold mountain air, and the temptation to stay in the cosy cafe would be too great. "Beware the chair". I gave myself a stiff talking to – no one else was going to do it.

"Get up you lazy git!" I said to myself, metaphorically kicking myself in the backside. I wearily got up from the chair, ignoring my complaining muscles, and set off up the hill at an easy jog-walk.

I kept to the grass verges where possible, in order to minimise the pain to my feet. Although I had confirmed they were not actually sides of raw beef when I had a quick look at them, they were certainly well tenderised.

As the sun came up, necessitating the stripping off of layers, hat and gloves, Martin came round the corner in his dark blue Mercedes convertible, one of the most welcome, if unlikely, ultra trail support vehicles I had ever seen. He waved several pairs of socks at me from the window, and yelled out words of cheerful encouragement. Stopping at a layby, within spitting distance of the mouth of the tunnel, he opened the boot of the car to display a veritable smorgasbord of treats – chocolate biscuits, fruit juices, Coke, dried and fresh apple and more! It could well have supplied an entire contingent of ultra runners, instead of the only entrant – me.

The combination of the sun, luxurious clean socks, and Martin's cheerfulness were infectious.

I took what I needed and carried on to the mouth of the tunnel. Martin was going to drive up to the lights and wait, whilst I chatted to the border patrol one last time to see if I could trot through, and to discover whether or not the Col had reopened.

Martin zoomed off and joined the series of hairpins that snaked up the side of the mountain to the mouth of the tunnel. I took a more direct trajectory – not so much a path as a scramble up a series of banks and retaining walls, waving to Martin every time I crossed the road. We were playing a curious game of tortoise and hare. I reached the border, and as expected the French guard said "Non" in no uncertain terms, and confirmed that the Col was impassable due to the "several metres of snow". As the children's book *We're Going On A Bear Hunt* says "If we can't go over it, we can't go under it, we can't go round it, we'll have to go through it".

17 March 2007, When In Rome

David and I stood in the shadow of the Colosseum in the heart of one of the oldest and most picturesque cities in the world.

It remains the oldest amphitheatre in the world and was a marvel of Roman engineering. I had seen it in pictures and movies, but it was even more impressive in the flesh.

In fact, the whole of Rome was amazing.

We had flown in the previous day after I had had a stressful week's work, travelling over most of the North of Italy meeting the management of a couple of corporations and site visits as part of a research project I was undertaking for various clients. I had spent a lot of time drinking coffee, eating biscuits and sandwiches from service stations – admittedly better quality in Italy than anywhere else I had been, but still of dubious nutritional value – and commuting hundreds of kilometres every morning and evening. I needed a break and was pleased to get a weekend pass from Mrs R to fly to Rome and see some sights as well as hang out with David. On top of that, I was actually meeting a sometime client, broker and friend, who had decided to run the marathon as well. He would be way ahead of David and me though, as he was trying to qualify for the Commonwealth Games team to represent the Isle of Man.

The Commonwealth Games is a bit like the Olympic Games, an international multi-sport event held every four years. The difference to the Olympic Games is that participants must come from a country in the British Commonwealth, such as Canada, Australia, England, Scotland, and many more from the old British Empire. There are 71 countries that qualify to send participants to the Games, and these include tiny states such as the Isle of Man.

The trip from the airport was an eye opener, and not only for the distinctive Roman driving style adopted by everyone including our cab driver. Before visiting Rome, I had had visions of a few unrecognisable artefacts painfully extracted from their graves by wizened volunteers using brushes as some building project or other uncovered another remnant from history. The reality was anything but. In amongst the industrial outskirts of a thriving modern industrial city, were Roman aqueducts and the remains of ancient buildings, some over 2000 years old. On the left there would be a drab concrete grey apartment block, and on the right there would be a beautiful, decorated ancient villa.

From the airport we went straight to the "expo" to check in, and queued for an age before being able to pick up our numbers and free cotton t-shirts. David had chosen Rome because it was six months after the Monaco Marathon and his failed attempt at breaking four hours. He had been able to carry his fitness, and had been hugely motivated to train despite the cold, damp or even snowy mornings to put in the required miles. I had been less than motivated in training as I had already achieved my goal, and was rudderless in terms of setting myself to a new and refreshing challenge. However, the euphoria of crossing the finish line had become like a drug to me, and I was more than happy to sign up for another, different, marathon with David. I had a dozen excuses for why my training had not been as thorough as it had been for the Monaco Marathon, but this was my fourth marathon and I was confident of finishing.

After the expo and wandering around for ages trying to find the tube station, and then my hotel, I was happy to collapse in reception and watch a rugby game on TV in the afternoon. Rome was exceptionally busy that weekend as St Patrick's Day was the same day as marathon day, and the Irish rugby team was playing a key Six Nation's tournament game against Italy, there in Rome. The day of our arrival Ireland had won the game with my hotel room situated one floor up from one of Rome's most popular Irish pubs. The Irish had won the game by a healthy margin, and the pub was predictably full to overflowing, with celebrations spilling out into the street. I had carried a lot of fatigue and stress in addition to my running kit from home, and was worried about getting a decent night's sleep, so went to bed early, with the window shut to muffle the noise. About half an hour later, I awoke with a dry mouth and covered in sweat. I opened the window to let in some air, the air-conditioning predictably non-existent.

Which made the noise phenomenal. It was like actually being in the pub, but without the fun. Or the Guinness.

I tossed and turned trying to block out the noise. I had some ear plugs, but I could still hear the crowd from the pub, even with my head tucked firmly under the pillow. It was no good; I had to close the window. An hour later, mouth drier than the Sahara, and lying in a pool of sweat, I got up to open the window. I lay in bed listening to the infuriating sounds of people enjoying themselves, and tried to force myself to relax. "Breathe deeply; in and out; relax the muscles; think about nothing". Angrily, I would turn over and start again. It was a long night until 3am, closing time for Rome pubs. As the last revellers faded into the background, I finally drifted off to sleep.

Ping! went my alarm. My eyes snapped open. It was 6am, but I was already awake.

Marathon day, and the first time I had had to take a shower before a race, but I needed it to get rid of the fatigue that was cloaked on me. I had grabbed breakfast, and made my way to meet David to dump our bags, and stretch before the start.

As David and I tried to keep warm on the shaded cobbles below the Colosseum, I was feeling very nervous. David was in fine form, having been extremely motivated for the race, and looked relaxed and well rested. Meanwhile, my sunglasses covered my bloodshot eyes and anxiety.

With immaculate Italian planning, the gun went off 20 minutes past 9, the 20 minute delay to allow for a glitch in the TV scheduling. Carried forward by 10,000 of our closest friends, we crossed the start line a couple of minutes later, and started jogging at an easy pace and enjoying the sights. David was chatting away, but within minutes the pace was faster than I was entirely comfortable with, and even though I had no electronic gadgetry such as heart rate monitor or GPS, I knew instinctively that the pace was a little high, as I was sweating and breathing far more rapidly than David, and early in the day.

The sleepless night and stress were put to the back of my mind, and David and I fell into a well practised rhythm.

We spoke about everything on our runs – training and the races. Life histories, experiences, girl friends, marriage, kids and jobs were all mulled over, thrown back and forth and dissected. It took our minds off the running, but was also an externalised version of what happened when I was running alone. I might have a sleepless night worrying about a certain issue at work, but once I had come in from my run a course of action was clear in my head. It was like opening up a box of Christmas tree lights to find a tangle of wire and bulbs; but whilst running I was able to untangle the mess in order to present a gleaming, uncluttered string ready for the tree.

We made our way past a few landmarks in Ancient Rome, and into the industrialised suburbs. Passing various aid stations, we would grab handfuls of orange segments and suck the juices out of them, hurling them into the large boxes provided for litter. David missed a box and hit a Policewoman entirely accidentally, on her back, leaving a splattered sticky mess on her jacket as she struggled to hold back the crowd. The police in Rome were as fascinating as the architecture – there seemed to be infinite different divisions – local, municipal, financial, carabanieri...the list went on. Every single one of them was immaculately turned out in their appropriate uniform, with highly polished Sam Browne belts and leather shoes. The female police wore their long hair down, and had liberally applied layers of make up on their faces. Designer sunglasses were obligatory. It was an interdepartmental fashion parade.

We enjoyed the camaraderie and sightseeing as we ran, but I was struggling from early on to keep up the pace being set by David. My breathing was becoming increasingly laboured, and at one of the crowded aid stations, as I slowed to grab a plastic tumbler of water, someone shouldered me out of the way and I lost my balance, partially twisting my knee in the process. I was angry and upset; I could feel my mental strength seeping away into the gutter with the water from the tumbler.

I kept my agony to myself and let David keep up his monologue. A couple of minutes after the aid station bumper cars incident, we ran past a competitor who, from his zombie-like gait, appeared to be struggling. The course had few hills, unlike Monaco, part of the reason David had picked it as it would be easier for him to reach his goal: to beat four hours. However, the course had a small but steep upturn right at the moment that our fellow runner was wrestling with his demons. Just as we passed, he lost his internal battle and collapsed at the feet of a medical crew. I looked back over my shoulder to see them cover him with a space blanket and attach an electrode to his forefinger. Pleased that he was receiving the appropriate attention, but shocked at what we had seen, we continued in relative silence – just the plod of trainer on tarmac and tinny hiss from others' earphones.

Like a flock of birds moving as one entity, we zigzagged through the industrial outskirts of Rome before trouping under a motorway flyover. The tunnel was dark and dank, and the only runner with enough energy – few and far between – was trying to boost his own morale and that of those around him, by singing a little ditty borrowed from the football terraces and encouraging everyone to join in. We had covered almost 33 km/ 20m, and I had had enough. The fatigue, patchy form, and knee pain had all conspired to mentally break me. I stopped at the lowest point of the tunnel to stretch my leg, and David looked over his shoulder questioning me? I waved at him to carry on.

I had not hit "The Wall" resulting in a bodily collapse, but I had hit a wall nonetheless. I was ready to get on the Sweeper Bus. Almost in tears, I began the gentle climb out of the tunnel at a walk with a pronounced limp. Emerging into daylight, I caught sight of a group of girls waving a British flag, there to cheer along some of their compatriots. They saw the GBR designation on my number, pinned to the front of my t-shirt, and they cheered me on. I lifted my head and was able to break into a very slow jog.

The last few kilometres of the Rome marathon are some of the most beautiful of any marathon anywhere in the world. Competitors pass the Piazza Navona, Spanish Steps, Trevi Fountain, Piazza del Popolo... if you have ever received a postcard from Rome, the picture on the front will have been taken in the last 5km/3m of the Rome marathon course.

I didn't see any of it.

I gritted my teeth and pushed on, walking a bit, running a bit. Everything around me became a blur, apart from the cobbles. Each cobbled section, of which there were many, was like an added torture, sending my ankles all over the place and stretching my aching muscles in different directions just to stay upright. With every step I almost gave up; my body was screaming out to my brain to just stop and sit down. I passed the 1km to go marker, and caught sight of the Colosseum from the rear.

Cruelly, we had to run almost a full lap of the Colosseum. After this, I crossed the timing mat and staggered to the kindly volunteers giving out the medals.

I had crossed the line in three hours, fifty eight minutes and change. I was completely gutted, physically and emotionally due to fatigue, disappointment at not keeping pace with David, and for being slower on a tougher course than my previous effort. I was also euphoric at crossing the finish line, probably because the pain could then stop. I was able to walk quickly to get my drop bag with a tracksuit top, change of t-shirt and medal, and I made my way to the Irish pub that had so disturbed me the night before. David and his friends had made it there before me and had lined up a Guinness for me in advance.

Despite the fact that I had finished my fourth marathon, and in a very respectable time, I was still gutted because I knew I could have done so much more. It was like the physical pain had just melted away, and I knew that it had all been in my mind. After an hour or two I didn't even feel that tired. I left David to his extra night in Rome and grabbed a taxi for another terrifying ride, this time to the airport, cheered by the sight of people still staggering across the finish line as we passed the course, a good two hours after I had finished.

I was able to fully reflect on what I had done wrong, and also set myself a new goal. David had beaten me by 10 minutes that day.

I had a new goal.

19 June 2014, End Of Part One

"There was no other alternative. Nothing else to do. Don't beat yourself up over it. Hell, it's only 3k, I mean what's that, out of 100 plus km you've come so far?"

"But I've let everyone down."

"Don't be stupid. Come on, out of the car. It's only another 10k to Limone, and all downhill."

Martin had driven me through the tunnel, across the border, and we were now in Italy. It was a glorious morning, the sun warming up the mountain air and picture postcard views of the mountains all around. My head had dropped as we passed through the tunnel, the Mercedes' suspension soaking up the ruts and bumps of the century old tunnel, as I luxuriated in the plush leather interior after a night of constant motion. I couldn't help but feel I had somehow cheated and that people would call me out on it after the event. I was, after all, attempting to complete the challenge for charity.

Martin was right, though.

I lifted my head, took a deep breath, and unfurled myself out of the comfortable car, gingerly testing how my battered feet and creaking joints felt after the brief respite. I had two choices: I could follow the narrow road as it snaked down the hill, or I could scale the crash barrier at the side of the road and follow the camber of the hillside until I hit Limone.

I must have resembled some demented old-aged pensioner as my limbs were so stiff I could barely lift them over the barrier. In fact, I actually sat down on the barrier first, and then swung both legs over by leaning back and pivoting until they were the other side. As I put my legs down, due to the ground on the downhill side being a lot lower, I almost lost my balance. I would have rolled the final 10km / 6m into town had I fallen!

After a few minutes, everything loosened up and the pain in my feet subsided, perhaps numbed by the renewed punishment. Every now and again my trajectory would take me across the series of switchbacks as I descended the hill. I couldn't quite see Limone but I was so close I could smell woodsmoke from the chimneys; fires had been lit as, despite the warm sunshine, the mountain nights could still drop well below freezing, to which the snow on the Cols in plain sight attested.

A little, battered, blue, stereotypical Fiat emergency braked in front of me on a switchback. Before it had even come to a complete halt, the passenger, a petite brunette with closely cropped hair, jumped out of the car and started yelling at me in Italian. To say my ability to speak Italian was limited would be an overstatement. I could just about muster a cappuccino in a cafe. At a push.

Frantically waving at me and coming closer, I thought she might have been asking for directions, or perhaps announcing some sort of emergency. I looked around to see if there was any evidence of impending avalanches, as the white and yellow meadow flowers swayed to and fro in the gentle mountain breeze.

I started to think I was hallucinating, after all I had been awake and in motion for over twenty four hours, having worked a full and busy day, and then run 100km / 60 miles over the Alpes Maritimes. The brunette was joined by the driver, similarly jabbering away in Italian at me, before he registered my complete bafflement and started to speak in staccato English.

"Ben? Cro Magnon. Pietro sent us. Tea? Biscuit?"

"Er, that would be lovely, thanks. Pietro sent you?"

I choked back emotions which started to boil up, exaggerated in their unexpectedness and by fatigue. "You are here for me? Is there anyone else running from Monaco?"

Both Luca and Sonia, these wild Italians, laughed.

They were volunteers helping Pietro organise the start of the Cro Magnon, and would also be helping out during the running of the race. Pietro had mentioned my solo challenge, and he had asked them to find me as I crossed the border to give me some moral support, as well as hot tea and Digestive biscuits, apparently a true Italian ultra runner breakfast.

It was about 9am and they had been driving up and down the various roads and trails for over an hour looking for me, unsure of how I would enter into Italy, given the inclement weather and customs. I had also, unwittingly, made things a lot harder for them by cutting through pastures and meadows, steering clear of footpaths as my vision became narrower and all I wanted to do was sit in some cold water and have some breakfast.

Truly buoyed by their generosity and good spirits, and warmed by the hot, black, sweet tea and a handful of Digestives, I continued.

They said, in faltering English with a lot of gesticulation, that they would be waiting for me in Limone. A couple of hundred metres later, I saw a sign for a mountain bike track which should lead me into the village. I ducked under the low hanging branches and had a glorious run through heavy woods, gently downhill, with lovely soft earth under my feet. Every few minutes I would glimpse evidence of human habitation, a hint of concrete here, a flowerbed there, parked cars.

I was so close that I started to salivate at the thought of a toasted Panini, mozzarella seeping out of the sides and congealing on the plate, a hot cappuccino with velvety frothy milk, chocolate sprinkles, and a chair.

Then I reached a train track. A single file mountain train track. I could see Limone on the other side, but I was the wrong side of the barrier. Behind me was nothing but a field, and the mountain bike track. There was a button to press, presumably to alert the signalman that I wanted to cross, so I pressed it. Perhaps a farmer would occasionally need to get a tractor into the field, and hence cross the tracks? Perhaps the mountain bike riders would circle back and ride from whence they had come? At any rate, how many trains could possibly pass through Limone?

I leaned nervously over the barrier, careful not to overbalance with the weight of my backpack and aching muscles, and I nearly got my head taken off by a narrow gauge goods train. The tantalising glimpse of Limone disappeared as my vision was filled with a blur of blue and grey. Impatiently I waited, and waited, and waited, shifting my gait as I tried, unsuccessfully, to get comfortable.

Five minutes after the train had passed, I was being cheered into Limone village by Sonia, Luca and another of their volunteer colleagues, Paola. In a mixture of French, Italian, English and a lot of hand gestures, I managed to get across my wish list. They, in turn, managed to negotiate with the newsagent to let me sit in the fountain in the little square outside his shop whilst they passed me several cappuccinos and a Panini, all surpassing my expectations. I had covered over 105km / 63 miles, as my little mountain bike track had actually added an extra 5km / 3 miles to my journey, more than outweighing the lift I had received through the tunnel.

I munched, pensive, in the freezing cold water, inspected my blistered feet, and wondered how on earth I was going to be able to turn around in a few hours and run back the other way, with the added pressure of time barriers and the sweeper, like the Grim Reaper, closing the course and collecting people's numbers if they could not keep up.

I hoped I hadn't set the bar too high.

14 October 2007, Happy Trails

"What's the matter? Are you hurt?" I shouted ahead to my friend and neighbour, Alex Wurz.

"No." A man of many words.

"So what's the problem?"

"Nothing. I'm fine. You go ahead."

I pushed harder on my knees with my hands to help me climb the steep slope, one foot occasionally slipping on a rock dislodged from the dirt, throwing me off balance. I squeezed past Alex, thorn bushes like walls on either side of the single track grazing my arms and legs.

We were about a third of the way in to the 16 kilometre Trail run of Gorbio, my first ever off-road run. (School cross country races around Knowle Park were merely just an excuse to have a sneaky Marlboro Light behind a bush). I was training for the Milan Marathon, and training hard, as I was racing against David's record time in the Rome Marathon earlier in the year. I had been criticised by some to even attempt to race another marathon in the same twelve month period, but invariably these were people who had never even entered a marathon let alone finished one. For Alex, off-road running was part of his training; he was a professional sportsperson having been a BMX world champion at 16 and since graduated to faster modes of transport. He had persuaded me to enter the Gorbio race, and as it fitted in nicely with the training schedule I had prepared from various books and the internet, I thought I would give it a go. At the least it would break up the monotony of hundreds of lonely kilometres on the road.

The start line saw lots of grizzled and surprisingly sturdy veteran off road runners, with their trail shoes and aging mud splattered Camelbacks. They were in stark contrast to the skinny, lithe marathon runners I was used to. There was very little in the way of refreshments in the race, with the terrain effectively climbing up a mountain, running along a ridge, and then sprinting down the other side back to the village of Gorbio. We gathered under the 300 year old elm tree in the town square, and then we were off.

Alex went off with the front runners, through the narrow and cobbled streets of the village, whilst I held back, pacing myself. The first kilometre or so was reasonably flat, but it soon got very steep and my experience of hills in races had been the relatively short "Hernia Hill" in the Monaco Marathon, child's play compared to what I was facing outside of Gorbio. I was therefore surprised to catch up to, and even overtake Alex, as we enjoyed the spectacular view over the glittering and blue Mediterranean.

"Nice legs."

A disembodied voice shouted at me, heavily accented. "Very strong."

I sped up. We had crested the top of the climb and were running along the ridge which was gently undulating and like running on a carpet. I hurdled over a tree root sticking out of the ground. I thought I had left a struggling Alex behind and was secretly feeling very pleased with myself, given his credentials. It was clear from his voice that he had, however, recovered and was hot on my heels. Too puffed out to speak, I concentrated on staying upright and trying to put some more distance between us.

I could still hear Alex's thumping footsteps as we reached the end of the ridge and the hand drawn arrow pointing us down an improbably steep path. If you could call it a path. It was more like a dried river bed – loose rocks and boulders, the slope so steep the path snaked its way down the mountain. I gingerly stepped onto a rock and immediately felt it slip down the hill, taking my legs with it. I landed heavily on my backside, but was able to throw myself back upright with the momentum. Alex was slipping and sliding down the slope too, but staying upright with the sure footedness of a mountain goat. I turned round to face the slope to negotiate a steep two metre drop, and used my hands to lower myself down, scraping my t-shirt upwards and grazing my stomach in the process. Alex got to the rock and jumped, flying over my head, to land two metres further down the path and disappeared around a bed. Little stones and bits of dirt hit me in the face, debris from his courageous (insane) leap; I was speechless.

I picked my way down the final (steep) third of the race and trotted across the line five minutes after Alex in a respectable time of 1 hour 40 minutes, and 77th out of 180 entrants. I had loved the experience – being on the trails and in the mountains was like going back to my childhood and charging about the woods with my friends playing at any one of a hundred different kids' games, usually based on either James Bond or John Wayne. It was also different than a marathon or road race –time pressure was missing. When I finished my first (and any) marathon the first thing anyone asks is what time did I do, no matter the weather or course, and the field of participants tended to be huge and impersonal. Entry fees could run into hundreds of Euros for the big city marathons, being as they were huge money making machines. The Gorbio experience was much more about bringing people into the village, challenging terrain, weather and quite literally pushing oneself over the edge into the unknown. For €12 I had received a race number, free t-shirt, and a piece of stale ginger cake and a Coke at the end. Excitement, nature, a fresh challenge, and all for a bargain basement price. Why hadn't I tried this before?

2 December 2007, Retaking The Crown

I lay on the dirty Milan tarmac absolutely spent, covered in a rustling tin foil blanket, my calf and thigh muscles spasming uncontrollably. It was as if I was still running, despite being prone on my back. Mrs R and Andy looked on, partly worried and partly amused, whilst they handed me Coke.

Despite the quite obvious pain, I was elated. I had trained hard and sensibly, with an objective in mind, and had more than achieved my objective. I had been quite open about it, that I wanted to beat David's Rome marathon time, and had travelled to Milan with that goal in mind. David had run three hours forty eight minutes and change, and I had crossed the Milan Marathon finish line in just over three hours thirty nine minutes. The last five kilometres had been pure mind over matter, as I forced myself to ignore my screaming muscles, and even when an impatient driver pulled out onto the course and I ran into the side of his car, I forced myself to carry on, undefeated. It often helped me to mentally dedicate a kilometre to my family, and when things got really tough I would just repeat a name. Kilometre 37 was dedicated to Emily, KM 38 to Alice, KM 39 to Izzy, and so on.

The key to my training had been to enter any and all races in the lead up. The trail race had been one such race, but I had also run the Great North Run again, and every other race I could find, generally with Alex Wurz (whom I privately called the Psychotic Mountain Goat, given his prowess at descending in Gorbio) or any other friends I could press gang to join me. I had found that not only had it helped me improve my speed - I would try much harder in a race than I would in a training run – but that it also gave me focus and a social activity that did not involve copious quantities of food and drink. Or if it did involve copious quantities of food and drink, at least I was earning them with a decent training session beforehand.

I had also been extremely sensible with my nutrition, cutting out junk food and alcohol even when out with clients in the last few weeks before the race, slimming down in the process. Not long before the race, I had been on a fabulous family holiday with lots of sleep and relaxation. The race itself coincided with a business trip, and I spent Thursday and Friday seeing clients and companies, before having a relaxing day of sightseeing with Mrs R.

That night a cold bath was a precursor to a fabulous dinner with copious quantities of food and wine. Mission accomplished.

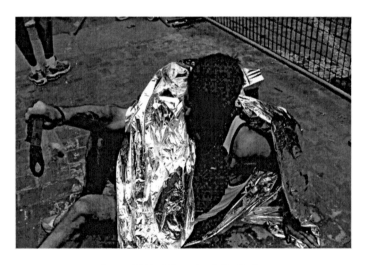

Rome 2010 - Photo by Sally Rolfe

25 February 2008, Uh Oh!

My leg muscles spasmed uncontrollably as I lost control of my bladder.

What the hell was going on? I put my hand on the slippery tiles in the shower to steady myself as the dizziness became overwhelming. My knees gave way as I collapsed into a heap in the shower tray, hot water cascading over me, making it hard to breathe. I crawled out of the shower, and shivering, opened the shower stall door. The changing room was empty, save for an overflowing laundry basket, towels dripping over the edge. I hauled myself across the deserted changing room floor, swiping the odd towel out of my way, my legs useless blocks of concrete. The heavy fire door had not been shut properly, enabling me to lever my fingers in between the gap and open it enough to manoeuvre my head and shoulders into the corridor. I could hear shouts, and footsteps rushing and then running towards me, and then nothing.

It was like looking through clouds. A glimpse of a blue and red uniformed Sapeur Pompier (paramedic) my hands and legs immobile. Pain. Lots of pain. Dom yelling something at me as I was wheeled past, screaming and writhing. I begged for a Coke. Then nothing. Bliss.

Pain and noise. Blue flashing lights. A phone ringing. The Sapeur Pompier questioning me, telling me not to sleep. In French.

Gradually the clouds dissipated, and I could hear lots of bleeping and whirring. I was attached to a drip and some monitors. Doctors and nurses came in and out, and once they saw I was awake started spoon feeding me baby food. It looked like baby food anyway, pale green and mushy. I started to feel better.

My legs relaxed, and instead of being made wholly of concrete they just had odd shaped lumps sticking out of them where muscles were cramping.

"What were you doing prior to your collapse, Mr Rolfe?"

"I had been to the gym. Running. On the treadmill." I looked down, and could see that I was naked apart from a hospital gown. Of course, I had been in the shower.

"I see." She made some notes on her clipboard. "And do you do much sport?"

"Yes. Quite a bit. I mean, I run marathons. I'm training for one now."

"And how far did you run this morning?"

"Er..." I was reluctant to say. The reaction I got from most people was one of incredulity at best, and accusations of irresponsibility or insanity at worst. "About 37 kilometres." I mumbled.

"37 kilometres? Really?"

"Yes." I said guiltily. She sighed as she wrote on her clipboard. I imagined she was making a note to check my head, as well as my body.

"I'm training for the Monaco Marathon. It's in a month. My friend..." I trailed off.

I had done it again. After my euphoric Milan experience, a friend had suggested we run Monaco in the spring, as he was raising money for a Zimbabwe charity. He had grown up there, and wanted to do something for the children, as the country was imploding. It was local, I could carry some fitness from Milan into the race. I thought how hard could it be?

"Mr. Rolfe, we have done some tests and we cannot find anything wrong with your heart, which is a positive. However..."

I was feeling a lot better, such that I felt I could even get up and walk, despite it being only an hour or two since my complete collapse. I was, however, feeling more than a little shaken up by the whole ordeal. The doctor's "However" was unsettling.

"However...your kidney function is very...erratic. It appears they were on the verge of complete failure. Have you taken any drugs?"

"No." I emphatically shook my head.

"Nothing? No alcohol?"

"No." Again.

"Ok. We will keep you in for a while to monitor your vital signs. Your blood is also showing signs of imbalances all over the place."

I was wheeled into the corridor and told to stay and rest, still attached to the drip and with a disconcerting footprint on the sheet that covered me. I wondered how and when that had got there.

Before my visit to the hospital, I was not aware of the effects long runs would have on my body. I had barely changed my nutrition strategy during runs from the Mentos and water that I had used with varying degrees of success since my first marathon, four years previously. I was also not aware that the body breaks down muscle tissue whilst running long distances, and the by product of this muscle metabolisation is toxic. The kidneys process this toxin and it passes out in the urine. Dehydration, poor nutrition and infections all exacerbate this condition.

The week before this fateful treadmill run I had been skiing for a few days with friends and family, arriving home the previous evening. It had been a busy week, getting three small kids to ski school at 8.30am every day, picking them up for lunch, skiing in between, and of course my diet consisting of beer and melted cheese. The friend with whom I was running the looming Monaco Marathon had accompanied us along with his family, and we had done some training whilst on holiday.

That ticked the poor nutrition and dehydration boxes.

Mrs R had heard from Dom that I was being carted off in an ambulance. As she ended that call, the phone rang immediately. It was one of my colleagues who angrily enquired as to why I was not in work that day. She was able to say that I was in hospital, but at that point she had no further details, and was greeted with apologetic silence on the phone. She confided to me later that she was equal parts worried and smug at the call.

On the way to the hospital, she had had to divert to the school to pick up Alice, who had been sent home sick.

That ticked the final box for a full house, explaining my collapse. I spent the next few days sick in bed, having made the virus that much worse, and a few days after that subjected to every single test known to man including allergies, blood tests, heart ultrasound scans, and a full body MRI. There appeared to be no long term damage but I added to my annual skin cancer check a blood test and thorough medical per doctor's orders.

I took away a number of different "learning experiences" from the episode: I always check my urine, especially during a long run, to see whether the colour was indicative of anything wrong. Generally, urine should be the colour of straw, and the darker it is the more I would need to drink. (You can also perform the same test through skin elasticity. Pinch the back of your hand and if the skin takes more than a second to snap back into place you are dehydrated.)

Secondly, I needed to pay more attention to my overall nutrition. I was pushing my body more and more, not getting any younger, and I needed to put back in what I was taking out. A few days later I got chatting with a fellow Dad at the bus stop as we waited for the school bus to pick up our kids. He travelled a lot but my wife and his wife knew each other through the kids. He had heard about my recent trip in the ambulance and he proffered a few tips. This particular father was a professional cyclist, World Champion and Olympic Gold Medallist Bradley McGee. Over time with his help I learnt what to eat at particular times, and the benefit of certain supplements such as protein. A race week diet plan was written for me, and which I learnt to follow slavishly, especially in the lead up to big training runs.

30 March 2008, Monaco Marathon

I staggered over the line in four hours, seven minutes and thirty seconds. The virus and trip to hospital had robbed me of fitness and resolve, and my final approach to the marathon had been dreadful. I was pleased to finish and draw a line under the whole experience, but it raised more questions than it answered. Just what was I actually capable of, with the right training and nutrition? I had actually posted a relatively respectable time for a notoriously difficult course (so difficult in fact that it would only ever have one more occurrence, in 2009, due to an explosion of flatter, faster races).

I also had unfinished business. I could not let that experience be my last marathon. I needed to go out on a high note. Just one more, and then I would stop running marathons (I told myself).

Saturday 5 April 2014, Normal, in Kent

"Daddy, everyone is checking their blood."

Alice was pricking her finger with the lancet, drawing a tiny spot of blood. She then put the drop onto her blood sugar meter, which would give her a number. This was something she would do every day around ten times, but pre-meals was extremely important as that would affect the amount of insulin she would need to inject, depending on the amount of carbohydrates she would consume during the meal itself. Everywhere we looked people were doing the same with a variety of different metres, and copies of "Carbs and Cals", our 'bible' for calculating the carb content of everything she ate, lay on virtually every table.

Alice was wide eyed, unashamedly staring. We had flown in the previous evening to join the Diabetes UK organised "Family Weekend". Nigel had told me about it, and he was one of the volunteers; most of the helpers were either Type 1 Diabetic themselves, or parents of children with Type 1 Diabetes.

Since Alice's diagnosis, her so called "Diaversary" [4] of 23rd December 2013, we had had a couple of months with very little support from the French system until we could find ourselves a slot in the middle of February. We had processed the stages of grief in isolation, but we had educated ourselves as much as possible in the meantime, with the help of Diabetes UK. In their own words, "Diabetes UK is the leading charity that cares for, connects with and campaigns on behalf of every person affected by or at risk of diabetes." [5] They had a terrific

---

4 "Diaversary" – the date on which the Diabetic was diagnosed. Some charities and action groups actually recommend celebrating the Diaversary, particularly that of a child, with presents and cake, so that a day with negative connotations can be turned into something with positive associations

5 From the homepage of Diabetes UK
https://www.diabetes.org.uk/About_us/What-we-do/

website of resources and information, people at the end of the phone to ask questions of, and even online forums where we could meet and discuss issues with other people going through the same experiences. Alice enjoyed (though often tentative and halting) conversations with other kids online through Diabetes UK.

We had pushed for Alice to be as open as possible about her condition and had to fight the education system which had a tendency to be very rigid, virtually brushing it under the carpet. We firmly believed that to learn about and maintain good control over her condition, she should be allowed to check her blood whenever necessary and as often as she liked, including during lessons if she felt the need. The system in place in the school was for diabetic kids to have set times, and to check their blood in the nurse's office only. This presented problems. If Alice felt woozy, her "danger" sign that she might be about to have a low blood sugar episode (hypoglycaemia or hypo), she needed to check her blood to confirm, and then treat it with a dextrose tablet or sip of Coke or Lucozade.

The school stated from the very beginning that in circumstances like that, Alice should excuse herself from class and head to the nurse's office to check her blood, treat the hypo and return to class when stabilised. This would entail her missing sizeable portions of class, risk alienating herself from her classmates and perhaps irritate her educators. It was, for us, a risk to her health. Hypos, as we had come to learn, were rarely dangerous if treated early enough, but if left untreated for even a short period could result in fainting, coma, brain damage and eventually death. On one occasion Alice had a hypo in the corridor when the nurse was dealing with a suspected broken ankle in the gym on the other side of the school.

Chatting to other parents and adults with Type 1, there were two very noticeable differences between the French and UK Health Services when dealing with Type 1 Diabetes. In our very limited experience in the French system, there was no hindrance about spending money or access to technology. However, there was very little in the way of educational resources or common support networks. Alice had been offered a pump immediately, and a couple of days later she had a working pump and a spare in case of breakdown, delivered to the door with a hospital appointment for several days to learn how it all worked. However, this approach seemed to take the view that we should deal with Alice's condition discretely so as not to offend anyone else with her perceived disability.

On the other hand, those we spoke to in the UK spoke glowingly about the education and support they were receiving, admittedly with the invaluable backup from Diabetes UK, but the NHS seemed to be very careful with the pennies, with two year waiting lists for a pump as the norm rather than the exception, and if it broke the patient would be back on injector pens whilst the pump was being fixed. Diabetes UK also played a big part with the public face of Diabetes, both Type 1 and Type 2. It was not something to be ashamed of, and there was no reason that a diabetic shouldn't lead a completely normal life, with a little extra in the way of admin, of course. For that reason they were campaigning to have a standard set of rights for Diabetics in schools, and educating the educators was part of that.

Consciously, we had taken on that role for Alice. The fund raising for my double Cro Magnon challenge had two effects: the first, of course, was raising much needed funds for Diabetes UK, but the second was to raise awareness of Alice's condition amongst her peers, parents, and teachers.

Our fund raising campaign had also gathered some local media attention, and the week before the Diabetes UK weekend, both Alice and I had been interviewed on the local radio station. We were in the studio for quite some time going over questions and answers, and in order to get our point across succinctly and precisely, there were plenty of stops and starts to the recording. Alice had been overawed as we walked in to the studio, a glass wall separating us and the DJ, and a huge bank of dials, switches and sliding knobs in front of us. Headphones on, Alice began falteringly, but as the interview progressed she grew in confidence, her answers increasingly eloquent and fluid as time went on. In the same way Alice's confidence in her life as a diabetic also grew over time, the local media attention helping get the message across without uncomfortable attention and ill-educated questions being levelled at her. Adult diabetics, people we knew socially, had quietly approached us and told us they too were Type 1 diabetic, something they had hitherto kept under wraps from all but their closest friends and family. More than one quietly expressed admiration for Alice and also for our welcoming and open attitude to the condition. Alice was learning that there was nothing to be ashamed of.

Alice became inspired by her own focus and was proud to be a source of inspiration.

The Diabetes UK weekend was a further eye opener for us. I had expected that we would have been one of the newly diagnosed families there, but people were tearfully admitting to a days old diagnosis. Some parents had multiple children with the condition. Other children had multiple conditions such as celiac disease and Downs Syndrome, to further complicate their lives.

It wasn't just Alice who was benefitting from experiencing a weekend with the condition totally normalised. These were people like us, volunteers and families alike, all getting together for a weekend of normality. Alice went to a safari park, and they had a disco for all the kids.

"Dad, what if I've forgotten something or run out of check-strips?"

"Darling it doesn't matter. Borrow one from Nigel, or one of the other volunteers."

"But what if I have a hypo?"

"Darling, I am sure that everyone on the trip will know how to treat a hypo [low blood sugar]."

The worry in Alice's eyes was reflected as concern and downright panic in the eyes of some of the parents when faced with the prospect of letting their children off for the afternoon in the care of other adults, people they had only just met. When I booked the weekend, I could not have imagined the effect it would have. Some parents had clearly never left their kids alone for more than a few minutes at a time, and we even heard stories of them getting up every two hours every night to check blood glucose levels. We, by contrast, were one of the more relaxed families, determined to live as normal a life as possible, and to demonstrate to Alice that there was no reason why she should not. The Diabetes UK weekend had a profound effect on everyone – parents, Type 1 kids and their siblings. Whether it was knowledge, newfound confidence, or just to know that we weren't alone with our daily challenges, it was a huge step in learning how to cope with living with Diabetes. Diabetes UK even offered the weekend to some at discounted rates, depending on their means, in order to help people attend.

Alice cried all the way back to the airport. She said she wanted to live her life surrounded by other Diabetics. Normally so stoic, her words were both touching and sad. She had clearly enjoyed the weekend (and it had been educational and supportive too), but she also just wanted to fit in and everyone to be like her if she couldn't be just like everyone else.

19 June 2014, Italian Hospitality

After some food and a long nap, some of which had been on a bench whilst I waited for someone with a key to open the apartment I had rented, I hobbled around Limone. My motives were twofold: to try and walk off as much of the lactic acid as possible and stretch tight muscles, but also to soak in the atmosphere. I had registered for many different races on several different continents, and in each case, large or small, I had felt at home.

I didn't consider myself an athlete. I counted Olympic Athletes and World Champions as my friends, but they were different. Every aspect of their lives was controlled, with time spent in laboratories analysing their gait and lung capacity. And they were paid for the pleasure and pain of participating in sport. Even when I went to championship ten kilometre races, the front runners would be professionals. Triathlons were a nightmare of hairless bodies with sub five percent body fat. I had to entertain clients, bring up a family and work fifty, sixty or more hours per week. I was hairy and had no idea what my body fat percentage was.

The start line registration "expos" of Ultra Trail races were like looking in a mirror. Everyone else was like me, there for the challenge, the buzz of pushing oneself to the limit, the love of the countryside and the mountains, (and probably to channel an addictive personality into something more constructive than destructive). Most people were hairy. Although, by the time the Cro Magnon came around I had been persuaded by a cyclist friend to shave my legs for a triathlon, and due to vanity I had continued to do so. My legs, if nothing else, had no body fat and were just muscles and veins. I liked that I had no hair to obscure their look.

Little by little, the cobbled, rambling streets of Limone were filling up with other Ultra runners (albeit those who had travelled to Limone by more conventional means such as car, train or bus). I recognised a few familiar faces, nodded hello, and then chatted to Luca, Paola and Sonia.

With a lot of hand gestures, plus a mixture of Italian, French and English, they very kindly extended me an invite to dinner at their accommodation that evening. Mistaking the invite to join them at the organisers' canteen, or a local restaurant, I accepted, and asked how I was to get there. I was told to wait where I had entered into Limone an hour or so earlier.

I stamped my feet and waved my arms about to stay warm. As soon as the sun disappeared the temperature plummeted, and having come into Limone on foot my choice of clothing was limited. Mrs R had dropped a little day pack off with a clean pair of shorts and a sweater, but I was certainly not prepared to be hanging around outside at altitude.

Not a moment too soon, the ubiquitous little Fiat screeched to a halt in front of me with Paola at the wheel. I had expected to meet all three of them there and to walk to a local eaterie or perhaps an organisers' canteen, so was a little taken aback. "In for a penny, in for a pound" I thought to myself as I got in and said hello to Paola in French.

Twenty minutes later we were navigating the tiny back streets of Limonetto, a neighbouring village, on foot, Paola having thankfully abandoned the car in a car park. I feared I may have added a few fingernail marks to the side of the passenger seat as she took the racing line through every bend without even a dab on the brakes.

We eventually reached a rustic Italian farm house. The bare wooden door opened, and I was welcomed in by Luca, Sonia, and Paola's husband. Far from it being a restaurant or canteen, it was actually the home of Paola and her husband. Sonia was busy cooking vast quantities of pasta in a huge cauldron-like saucepan, and some sort of beef stew in another. Luca was chopping vegetables for a salad. Paola's husband was laying the table in the middle of it all. Overhead hung a cloud of steam. They all seemed to be simultaneously shouting at each other over the din of sizzling. Hands were waved to emphasise the point, complete with knives and spatulas. Grateful to take the weight off my weary legs, I collapsed into a chair, and watched the interplay with a smile.

Even though it was hard to communicate, somehow we managed it during that meal. I managed to eat my own body weight in everything that was offered, declining to wash it down with beer or Chianti, preferring to stick to water. Paola's husband was a medic and Sonia a massage therapist, and much was made of inspecting my feet, complete with popped blisters (I had made the most of my downtime in Limone), and rubbing some lactic acid from my calves.

As Paola attempted to break the speed record for cars with a sub one litre engine capacity on the way back to my lodgings, I looked back at the magical evening I had spent with these incredibly generous strangers. If I had known I was going to someone's house, I would have taken at the very least a bottle of wine or some chocolates or flowers as a gift, but they had not asked anything in return from me. It typified the type of people that surrounded the sport of ultra running. I felt truly at home, and knew I would return the favour were it ever asked of me.

New Year's Eve 2008, Monaco

"Getting a fix of energetic stupidity has a downside. Like a junkie you need another hit soon, and it has to be bigger, better and harder than the last one."

I kept coming back to this line, an extract from *Life on the run: Coast to Coast* by Matt Beardshall. I had just finished reading the book that Mrs R had placed under the Christmas tree for me a few days earlier. I had not been able to put it down.

After the post training run collapse and visit to the casualty unit at Monaco hospital, Brad was helping me with my nutrition. In fact, he had seen me on the school run a few days after the incident, noticed my haggardness and pallor, and virtually insisted he teach me a thing or two. In November 2008, he had accompanied me on his bike, as I attempted to secure a personal best marathon time at the inaugural Nice to Cannes marathon. I missed my 2007 Milan marathon time by seconds, despite the Nice marathon being a lot less flat, and had been thrilled. In the meantime, I had also started running a lot more trail races with Psycho (Alex), partly for training but also because I loved them. I was becoming a junkie, but like a junkie, the fix needed to be bigger, better and harder.

A few days prior to Christmas, a former colleague, client, and friend rang me and suggested we run the Marathon Des Sables (MdS) together. The MdS was definitely on my bucket list, but I balked at the challenge. Six marathons in seven days across the Sahara Desert carrying all one's own kit and food was akin to running before we could walk, particularly as the furthest my buddy had run was a ten kilometre cross country race in Kent where he lived. I had suggested we run the Neander Trail as a warm up, see how we got on, then if it went well put our names down for the MdS.

The Neander Trail was a 50 kilometre ultra marathon across the mountains from the Col de Turini in Italy to the beach at Cap D'Ail just outside Monaco. The Col de Turini had been made famous as one of the trickier stages in the Monte Carlo Rally, often several inches under snow. It had actually been one of the very first Alpine ski resorts, although not used as such these days, there were still a couple of chair lifts in existence.

To make things more complicated, the start time of the Neander Trail was scheduled for 8pm, on Friday 6 June 2009. This meant that runners would be crossing tricky mountain trails almost entirely in the dark. The start of the Neander Trail was slated for almost the half way point of its big brother, the Cro Magnon.

Three of us duly entered the Neander Trail, improbably securing three out of the one hundred places in a hotly contested ballot, and were biting our nails fretting about how on earth we were going to train for a mountain ultra marathon in the dark.

Unwittingly Mrs R had provided me the answer wrapped up in shiny paper and a bow. Matt's book was a memoir of his charity run from one side of the UK to the other along the fabled Coast to Coast path, made famous by Wainwright a hundred years' previously. Matt had gotten a group of like minded friends together, recruited back up drivers to carry luggage and food, and completed the challenge raising money for Children in Need in the process. Matt had been injured in training, and relied upon the services of an ultra runner in Mexico called Dr "Mad Dog" Mike Schreiber to recover from the injury, and to reach the start line of his personal challenge injury free.

A few mouse clicks later, and I too was part of the "Mad Dog Online Training Team", and about to embark on a series of adventures, each bigger, better, and harder than the last.

4 June 2009, Triple Whammy

"You're deluded, by the way."

"Do what? What do you mean I'm deluded?"

"To do what you're doing. This weekend. Putting yourself at risk, like that. You've got a job and a family. You're deluded. Stupid. You shouldn't be doing it. What if you get injured? Or dead? What then?"

I was two days out from the biggest sporting challenge of my life, and I had been rendered utterly speechless by someone I had hitherto thought was one of my closest friends. In my head I knew that without any sport the likelihood was I would have had serious and long term health issues long before 2009. Due to my lifestyle changes I would probably live longer and was also enjoying life a lot more.

But he did have a point. There are, of course, inherent risks to any sporting endeavour. People are injured and even die every year while horse or bike riding, playing rugby, hockey, basketball or cricket. I had even heard, during a stint backpacking in the Antipodes, that lawn bowls had the highest fatality rate of any sport in Australia. Something to do with the heat and the demographic of the participants.

However, having run several marathons and a large number of shorter races both on and off road, I hadn't really considered that the Neander Trail, 50 kilometres across the mountains at night, would be any more dangerous than any of those. I was trained and equipped, both physically and mentally, for pretty much every eventuality. Of course, something could happen out of my control, such as weather or a broken leg, but then there are risks crossing the road.

In the time it took to have a quick coffee, a friend had managed to severely undermine my confidence. Perhaps particularly so, as it came on the back of a very tough time professionally. The subprime crisis had hit in earnest late in 2008, and my client base had diminished by two thirds from December 2008 to June 2009. I had been working harder than ever to rebuild my revenues, but it was like pushing water uphill. The Neander Trail had saved my sanity, giving me something to look forward to and focus on, other than the devastation that greeted me daily in the office.

The previous day I had received word that a business I had invested a large part of my savings in with a friend had folded, resulting in the loss of all my capital. I had hoped that this new enterprise would cushion some of the blows that the economic downturn was raining on my existing business.

The only thing that was keeping me sane was sport.

I had purchased a bike in the January sales and started cycling for cross training but with one eye on the Monaco Half Ironman triathlon later that year. It was the first time I had been on a push bike since my second hand purple Raleigh Chopper in 1984. I had written off that bike spectacularly, but was enjoying my MAMIL (middle aged men in Lycra) experience once I had worked out the gears and pedals!

I was taking some swimming lessons with the same goal in mind. Whilst I was working harder than ever, my reduced client base was not in the mood to be entertained, and I was making the most of the extra hours, putting the extra personal time to good use rather than sitting and brooding in the local Irish pub.

Race week rolled around, and I was doing my best to taper off from training and channel my nerves into carb loading and resting. The triple negatives made relaxing all the harder; to say that I was having a bad week was an understatement. All I could do to keep it together was focus on the job at hand.

6 June 2009, Neander Trail

Jesus, it was cold. Really cold. I wore every layer I had brought and I was still cold. There was a tiny wooden cabin, more of a hut really, and every person there, perhaps 300 or so including the volunteers, was queuing for one of the two loos. When my turn came I made my visit as short as I possibly could to minimise the unpleasant aroma assaulting my nostrils, then went back outside.

Everywhere I looked people were shoving great globules of Vaseline down the front of their Lycra tights, up their t-shirt tops, down the back of their trousers. People were taping up their feet to the point of mummification, and then putting Vaseline over the top.

An aura of excitement hung over the mountain top along with a thick, wet mist.

"Ouch! Oi, mind where you put that would you?" I turned around, rubbing the spot on my thigh where I had been jabbed by a ski pole. I was confronted by three Action Men types in French Foreign Legion tracksuits.

"Huh?" One of them said to me, with a less than friendly expression on his face.

"Er, never mind, it doesn't matter," I said as I took note of the scar running down one side of his face, exaggerating the frown on his lips. I looked down at his hands. A complete absence of paper cuts, but evidence of a tough life with tight white jagged lines across his knuckles, almost fluorescent in contrast to the deeply tanned skin.

I sidled away. My knowledge of the Foreign Legion was limited to the fact that it was an elite unit of the French military, shipped out to do the toughest jobs the French military needed done. Cracked lips and sand always sprang to mind whenever anyone mentioned them. They were typically based in North Africa in the old French colonies of Algeria and Morocco. However, the "Foreign" bit of the name referred to the recruitment of non-French nationals, and after a pre-agreed time in service, with an honourable discharge, a retiring Legionnaire would be afforded a French passport. This often gave rise to the rumour that the major motivation of those joining the Legion was to run away from something in their own country, and able to start afresh in France after serving in the military. Doomed romantic liaisons or questionable police records were often proffered as reasons. Whatever the background of my fellow trailers, I was not about to start a fight with one over a ski pole accidentally jabbed into my backside.

I wasn't really nervous about the task ahead, I just wanted to get started. I had been nervous in the lead up, but with Mad Dog Mike in my corner I was confident in my training, and with Brad's nutrition and cross training help my body shape had changed. I had muscles where previously I had had none, and was about to take the start line of the Neander Trail healthy and injury free. Mad Dog had also helped my with my kit selection; he had encouraged (demanded) that I take as little as possible. For nutrition I merely had some chopped apple and a protein enriched flapjack called a Go Bar - that Brad used on the bike. I had two litres of very diluted Isotonic powder and some spare powder in my pack. I had the compulsory kit of Gore Tex jacket, running over jacket, long sleeved technical t-shirt, and some Lycra tights. I also had gloves and an Ali G style beanie cap which was supposed to be quick drying and warm. I wore my normal running shoes at Mad Dog's recommendation, given most of his ultra trail experience in the 70's and early 80's was done in Asic Tigers or Dunlop Green Flash. Most of my kit had been picked up on special offer in the January sales, including my twenty Euro backpack. The contrast in cost between trail races and triathlons had never been more evident, with triathletes spending many thousands on bikes and wetsuits. [6]

Two of the three of us that had entered together had taken the bus up to Col de Turini earlier that day. The Cro Magnon had been cancelled due to snow lying on the higher mountains, and even though the Neander Trail did not reach nearly such a high altitude, we had been promised snow too. The Cro Magnon entrants had mostly decided to do the Neander Trail instead, which made the field bigger, much more competitive, and a little crowded, at least at the start.

I imagined that the sun had started to go down, as the fog precluded any hint of sun. The sky started to get even darker, and not a moment too soon we were off. This was unlike any other race I had been in, even some of the trail runs. Only the first couple of people ran. The course set off up a steep hill punctuated every ten or fifteen metres with a pylon carrying the chair lift. After about 50 metres of altitude gain, there was snow, previously hidden from view by the low clouds.

The grass under foot had been wet and slippery, making progress up the steep hill even harder. My gloves were already muddy from steadying myself as I slipped and slid. Once we hit the impacted snow, the lack of traction became even worse; I tried to stay upright, looking like a demented Bambi on ice. To add to my woes, the

---

[6] I was already in the process of training for my first triathlon when I took the start line of the Neandertrail in 2009. I had purchased an aluminium low cost roadbike for about €900 in the January sales, and what with tri suit and entry fees had spent more than €1000 for the race. I was lucky in that my wetsuit, shoes and pedals (themselves worth Euro200-300 each!) I managed to borrow from friends. Contrast that with my trail running, and races can cost as little as Euro15-20; the shorts were Lycra undershorts and cost around Euro10 from the local sports superstore; the t-shirt was a race shirt that I got free for completing another race. In fact, the highest costs were my normal running shoes, Euro150 if I didn't buy them at sale time, and the Gore Tex jacket which was a Christmas present but probably cost Euro100 or so. I am still using the jacket 6 years and many ultra marathons later. The bike is long gone in favour of an even more expensive carbon fibre model!

route was single file and people were trying to get past from behind me, whilst those in front got slower and slower. Those with the trekking poles seemed to have better balance, but they were twice as difficult to pass safely, errant poles poking bullseye bruises to my shins, adding to the one on my derriere I had picked up before the race had started.

Thankfully, the path ended, the mist cleared a little and I could see the trail snaking down the side of the hill until it reached a cinder trail. I decided to follow another runner and take the shortest possible route down, most of it on my backside, grabbing at clumps of grass and trying to avoid the hairy sheep grazing unconcerned.

The initial chaos of the start well and truly behind us, runners were able to find their own pace, competitors stringing out in a loose line. Some sprinted off into the distance and others dropped back. My main concern was not getting lost as the sun set. We headed up another climb, ending in a ridge which we followed closely, steep drop offs flanking both sides. Dusk gave way to night, the fog lifted, and it became easier to follow the course as I latched on to other headlamps in the distance. As the ridge smoothed out there appeared to be no path at all, and there were no banners or signs declaring which way to go. A party of three runners a few hundred metres ahead of me, including the lead woman, fanned out and descended the slope on all three sides. A few minutes later, garbled Italian shouts echoed from the left of the ridge, happily coinciding with my arrival at the invisible junction. His comrades rejoined him, and I tucked in just behind.

One of the key aid stations marking an approximate half way point was Sospel, nestled in a valley next to a river. The female leader and her group had long since left me in their dust as I ran down the trail which gave way to the paved road entering Sospel. A couple of kilometres before the refreshment stand, as I could hear the strains of loud music drifting up the hillside, I was joined by a phalanx of fireflies. My legs were moving fluidly, a far cry from my first painfully slow trail descent where Psycho had flown over my head. It was like being in a fairy tale, both magical and unreal. Something clicked inside my head, and I knew from that moment I was hooked. I knew in that moment that this would be my first of many trail ultras.

The air temperature was noticeably warmer in Sospel, and I took the opportunity to shed a few layers, grab a couple of handfuls of chopped apple from my pack, refill the bladder with water and powder, and then run out the other side of the village. Plenty of other runners were taking advantage of the chairs, receiving massages from their friends and family or official team crews. I decided there would be plenty of time for that at the finish.

A series of climbs and descents merged into one another as I fought through my fatigue. Any sensible sane individual would be tucked up under a nice warm duvet but for some reason I was running along mountain trails in the middle of the night. It wasn't always easy to keep a positive sense of humour, particularly when the batteries on my headtorch packed up. It took a tree route and a tumble for me to realise that they weren't actually giving much light at all. I had a spare headlamp with fresh batteries in my back pack but I was struggling to find it in the dark, so I decided to change the batteries in mine.

Big mistake.

My cold hands fumbled and I dropped one of the batteries. I had to wait an age for another runner to reach me. I flagged him down, and once he had recovered from the shock of being accosted by a big hairy thing in the dark, I borrowed the light from his headlamp to retrieve my errant battery.

A couple of kilometres later, I was stopped by another runner, an aged Italian competitor, who was suffering from the same problem. His batteries were completely dead and he couldn't see to fix his torch. I stopped, without being asked, to shine my light while he located and replaced his batteries. The spirit of trail running, so different to uber competitive road races, was never more starkly emphasised to me. Since that moment I have been a firm believer in trail karma, and rather than ticking off rankings or elbowing past on a narrow path, I will always offer assistance and support. One never knows when one is going to need it oneself.

As I meandered our way through various villages, getting closer and closer to Cap D'Ail and more familiar to me from various local trail races, my headlamp picked out the insignia of the Foreign Legion on two runners ahead. They were walking, clearly suffering. I caught up with them and to my surprise one of them initiated a friendly chat. The third member of the team had gone ahead, racing for a podium place, and these two were just trying to get to the finish. The friendly one was French and lived with his wife and children in La Turbie, a couple of kilometres from the finish, when he wasn't on posting with the Legion. The other, quiet and unsmiling, was from Bulgaria and didn't speak much French let alone English. I quietly wondered about his story and the rumours about foreigners joining up for the protection and anonymity. Even though they could barely communicate with each other, there was clearly a bond and an understanding between them, perhaps bred from shared experiences. In any case I had no doubt about their ability to finish the race and I left them behind me.

I emerged from some trees to see the picture postcard view of Monaco far below me. I was on the windswept Mont Agel, next to the bubble like radar station. I was wandering about the summit in a state of confusion, fatigue clouding my sense of direction. I was concerned, but not particularly panicking, because I knew I could get to the finish, but perhaps not by the path of the Neander Trail.

I had obviously missed a marker, and was technically lost.

New movements became increasingly erratic, my decision making ability affected by fatigue. A few minutes after arriving at the fort, I was joined by another runner, also lost. Together we backtracked to find the missed junction, and after retracing about a kilometre, we could see a snake of headlamps far below us. Rather than backtracking even further, we decided to run down the side of the mountain, taking care not to trip and somersault down the hill, until we reached the sheep track cut into the side of the hill.

As I reached the stony beach at Cap D'Ail, and jogged up the red carpet to the finish, the first rays of sun shine were bleaching the dark horizon.

I was an ultra runner!

I caught up with all three Foreign Legionnaires in the canteen the organisers put on for all the finishers and volunteers in the sailing school at Cap D'Ail. We munched on a selection of pasta and ham and cheese sandwiches, and toasted our relative successes in several different languages with non-alcoholic beers (the French Legionnaire was particularly miffed at the lack of a proper drink with which to toast our achievement, but non-alcoholic beer was all the organisers had provided).

In striking contrast to my previous runs, the camaraderie of the experience was never more evident. We had little in common (not even language!) other than the previous few hours on the trail. We had all been in it together. No one hesitated to support another runner, giving a little bit of a morale boost where and when necessary. I was reminded of my first Rome marathon when I was pushed out of the way of the refreshment stand by a competitor and almost fell.

I stayed to the very end, and got a lump in my throat when the winners clapped the last finishers over the line. The whole event had been very moving for me. The previous week's business difficulties had been slotted into perspective. A newfound sense of confidence and peace washed over me.

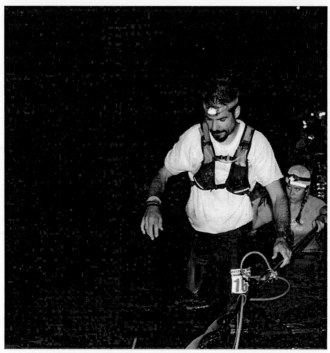

**River Crossing, WS100 2013, Best Pacer Chloe Romero just behind
- Photo by Keith Facchino, Facchino Photography**

Saturday 20 June 2014, Cro Magnon

It all seemed very familiar. A dark, cold, bleary-eyed 4am.

In the mountains. Nervous excitement. The smell of Deep Heat, sweat, and Vaseline. Three men wearing tights and headlamps lined up against a wall having a last minute pee.

A couple of months earlier I had been huddled under an awning with 25 strangers trying to shelter from a rain storm before the start of a 45km trail run. A month before that I had been in Barcelona for a marathon. Four years before, I had been on the very same start line for the 2010 edition of the Cro Magnon, my first attempt at anything over 100km, and more than double the distance of my previous longest Ultra, the Neander Trail.

The nerves were the same, uncertainty hovering in my thoughts. Was it even possible? Four years previously, it was just the Cro Magnon. Like the addict I had become, my search for the running high had grown more and more ambitious, and this was my "return journey", having run over 100km to the start a day previously.

What on earth had I been thinking? My feet had barely recovered from the pounding they had taken on the way up to Limone, and I still had blisters despite having popped them several times already. The skin underneath was so damaged, they just kept coming back. It was only then that the hard realities of my previous Cro Magnon filled my thoughts, memories of just how hard it actually was to finish.

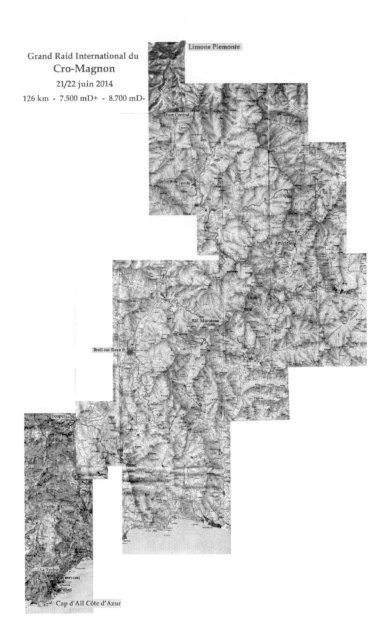

Grand Raid International du
Cro-Magnon
21/22 juin 2014
126 km - 7.500 mD+ - 8.700 mD-

19 June 2010, Cro Magnon

My tongue was the texture of sandpaper and twice its normal size. I sucked as hard as I could on my Camelback hose, each drop like nectar. I was covered in sweat, drops soaking the dusty floor as I trotted onwards. The sting of the grazes on my knees were subsiding, and I felt rather than heard the sound of another runner behind me.

"Ca va?" he said as he thundered past, turning his head to look me in the eyes.

"Oui." I replied unconvincingly.

I refused his offer of help, the rules of the race state that runners should be entirely self-sufficient, except at designated aid stations, and after having trained for months I was determined to finish unaided so as not to be disqualified. I steeled myself, trotted on, the sun beating down and the dust from the other runner drying my mouth even further.

It was almost 1pm, and I had been on my feet since 5am that morning: pre-dawn, setting off from the slightly chilly Limone Piemonte – a ski resort - in the Italian Alps. The route would take me to the finish – to the town that was twinned with Limone, Cap D'Ail in France. The two towns are perfectly juxtaposed, with Cap D'Ail a small beach resort favoured by royalty of the landed and Hollywood variety on the Cote D'Azur, bordering the fabled town of Monaco. In the meantime, runners encountered 5900 metres of altitude gain, and 6900 metres of descent on the way, most of it technical, following the old Spice Route. The path took in impressive mountain forts (how on earth did all those bricks find their way up the mountain?) that saw heavy action in World War Two, World War One and even before, with the debris of warfare gently eroding away under the elements. I saw tanks, 19th Century cannon, and other remnants of the darkest periods in recent history. That was not where the history stopped, however, as the run received its name from the discovery of some of the earliest man made markings found in France, and the concept of the Cro Magnon was born.

I had decided to enter the run because to qualify you needed a "point"; points could be gained with a trail run finish of 50km plus, with 2500 metres of positive altitude change and descent. The Neander Trail finish had not only given me my point, but also one of my most treasured memories running down into Sospel alone in the dark, just the moon, headlamp, and fifty fireflies floating weightlessly around me.

I decided to enter the Cro Magnon to raise money for Cancer Research UK again. Mad Dog Mike was enlisted to help me with the training schedules, and Brad helped me with nutrition, whilst Psycho was there for training runs and speed work. I was having a blast in training, learning new techniques and about my body. It wasn't always easy, getting up before dawn, the pain of hill sprints, the boredom of solitary long runs, but I knew that in the end it would be worth it. Not to mention the fun of completing two marathons and a 45km/28 mile ultra trail race as part of the training.

Race day was party day. All the preparation, training, nutrition and focus were forgotten. The start was at a chilly 5am. Limone was an old town, the streets too narrow for cars. 400 competitors plus associated supporters and race volunteers meant that we set off as one seething mass slithering through the damp streets. The pack soon thinned as we emerged from the village onto the meadows – which in the winter would have been the nursery slopes of the ski resort. We climbed uphill with the peloton shedding people as quickly as I was shedding clothes and putting them into my pack.

The sun came up, highlighting the beautiful mountain views. If I had much breath to give, puffed after the long climb as I was, the views would have taken it away. I lost a few seconds every time I paused to stuff something in my back pack, but at least this enabled me to admire a landscape I would never have otherwise seen. Despite the hardships inherent in such a challenge, I felt truly lucky that I was experiencing something that so few others will ever see.

After what seemed an interminable ascent for several hours, we turned off a glorious meadow carpeted with mountain wildflowers, and set off up a "dried out" river bed. There was ice and snow in the bottom of the narrow couloir. The gloves and hat went back on.

Once I emerged from the river bed (on my hands and knees) the sun was fully out and the sky that glorious blue that you only see in postcards, without a single cloud. I was struck by how quiet everything was – no traffic noise, no phones, no people, just a couple of mountain crows surfing thermals above me. I am sure that I was smiling as I broke into a jog. Before long we reached the Forte Centrale that I had previously only skied past. This marked the border between Italy and France; fortunately no passports were required (although the rules stated that we had to carry photo identity cards of some description in case there was a border check).

Almost immediately after the fort, we climbed single file up another peak, and whilst one could be forgiven for looking forward to some flat or downhill afterwards - it was a traverse around yet another mountain but snow covered the path – the ground was like an ice rink turned by 45 degrees, so I had to waddle, crab-like without grace, to the right in order to counteract the constant effect of gravity towing me to my left.

The event was held at the time of the full moon in June, thoughtfully chosen to aid the night sections with the best chance of moonlight and the weather at its most clement. Despite this timing, snow and blistering heat were often both encountered. Marco Olmo, the Italian ultra trail legend, had won the Cro Magnon a record six times, along with a host of other events such as the Ultra Trail of Mont Blanc. The previous winner of the race before my undertaking was Dachhiri Dawa Sherpa, another winner of the UTMB. The Cro Magnon, whilst less than a quarter of the size of the UTMB in terms of field size, was certainly taken seriously by the ultra running community at large.

I tried to put aside the seriousness of the race, and concentrated on enjoying it, walking up steep sections per the Mad Dog training plan, and Boy were there some steep sections! The race took in 5900m of positive altitude change, quite a lot of it in the first half. One particularly difficult section was a very steep couloir which had been strewn with man sized boulders after a recent avalanche, trees so old that I couldn't wrap my arms round the trunks, the tops having been snapped off like toothpicks by the force of nature. I climbed up, slowly but surely, having worked hard on my upper body and core strength in training. I noticed some other runners were making their way back down the way they had come having been beaten by the Cro.

As the course slowly descended, in hap hazard fashion towards the coast, the sun and the mercury both rose. I was filling up my Camelback with two litres of fluid at every aid station, adding my electrolyte powder every time, and yet it was taking me less and less time to empty it. I was running with another participant through an achingly beautiful meadow, past a mountain lake, and instead of taking in the view, I got down on my hands and knees and drank from a feeder stream. I tried in vain to put some into my Camelback.

Not long after, we traversed a valley, another steep drop off to the left, and a narrow sheep path cut into the turf. I followed the markers along the path, running solo, and lost my footing as fatigue and dehydration began catching up with me. I slid for ten or fifteen metres down into the valley before I could stop myself, and haul myself back up to the sheep track, thankfully with nothing more than a few cuts and grazes.

I encountered another runner, who while thundering past me, asked me if I was ok. The camaraderie almost brought a tear to my eye; it was a far cry from people pushing and swearing at aid stations in the big city marathons. It was all I could do to push myself onwards to the next aid station, and that was only half way point!

At Col de Turini, made famous by the Rallye de Monte Carlo as one of the most technical stages, and one of the original Alpine ski resorts, the organisers of the Cro had laid on a very well stocked aid station. My practise was to have a protein and energy bar, and some chopped apple, very kindly provided by my enthusiastic crew: Dom, Paul, Martin, and Mark. However, the first thing on my mind was water, Coke, energy drinks, anything liquid. I sat down and drank. Once my thirst was slated, I concentrated on forcing down a Go Bar, although some runners were tucking into full meals of soup, bread and pasta, with cake and chocolate pudding! Armed with my friends' wisdom and my own experience, I knew that my stomach couldn't cope with much more than a small snack, the blood being used elsewhere in my body as I ran. Besides which, whatever they were putting into themselves, they would have to carry up the next hill.

Not wanting to hang around, I set off down the road after only a few minutes. After reaching a family picnicking a couple of hundred metres from the aid station, they directed me back to the tiny little path that led into the woods, and the second half of the Cro. The Neander Trail would start from that aid station in a couple of hours, so I was aiming to get a decent head start.

The route was a lovely wooded path, gently undulating for the next 10km/6 miles or so, and I spent the time with a runner, but not a participant. He was actually a medic, drafted in from a bit further down the coast to Marseille, to run a certain section of the course, for fun, but to check out runners and administer medical attention if necessary. Once again, the organisers impressed me by seemingly thinking of everything. He carried a high powered walkie talkie, and over the crackle of his radio I heard the gun go off to start the Neander Trail. They had started this race a bit earlier than previous years, to give participants a better chance of navigating the trickier sections in daylight.

Emerging from the woods, we were greeted by a World War One vintage tank next to a decrepit bunker – perhaps part of the fabled Maginot Line, which lined the border between France and Italy after the First World War to prevent a Nazi invasion. It was fascinating to see all the history before my eyes, yet another of the many sights I would never have otherwise set eyes on, except perhaps in an A Level History textbook or black and white movie or news reels. My aching body was temporarily forgotten as I daydreamed about the story of the people who had abandoned the tank in that spot, making it a permanent marker.

As I descended into Sospel, it was approaching dusk. The previous year, my descent (from a slightly different angle) had been in the dark and accompanied by fireflies. This time I was dropping down into the valley in daylight. My quads were screaming. I was so grateful for all the extra quad training that Mad Dog had put me through, as I think I would have been a DNF (Did Not Finish) if I had not had it, at that point. Brad, my cyclist friend, met me 1km before Sospel, as it was a public footpath, and we walk / jogged to the aid station. I loaded my Camelback with fluids, had some apple, and set off almost as soon as I had arrived. I was aware that the next leg was brutal, remembering the climb out of Sospel on the Neander Trail.

I walked up most of the hill with my hands on my knees helping my forward motion like pistons. The climb was every bit as brutal as I had remembered, with the added bonus that I had already been on my feet for over twelve hours. Night would be falling soon, and I was starting to flag. I was thirsty, but I had mistakenly added too much powder to my Camelback, and the sweet taste was making me gag. As I emerged above the tree line, the climb stretched above me, seemingly endless.

A long haired Italian buckled in front of me, his knees just gave way, and he collapsed into a heap on the floor, his eyes welling up. I asked him if he was ok – in French, and if he needed a drink or some food, but he declined. He was facing his own demons, as I had faced mine earlier, and there was nothing more I could do for him. Perhaps he would pull himself together and finish, perhaps his race was over. I made a mental note to inform the next marshal I saw to satisfy the trail running karmic gods, and left him. I knew that the marshals wouldn't leave him on the trail forever, and it wasn't as if I had the strength to carry him.

My competitor's discomfort in a strange way made me stronger. Perhaps it was determination, stubbornness, something to prove to myself, or merely saying a few encouraging words out loud to him had had the effect of encouraging me too, but I continued the climb a little quicker than before.

I emerged onto a flat section, still barely in daylight, but I was flagging – badly. I saw Brad, who had mountain biked in to give me a boost, and he pointed me in the direction of a standpipe for livestock, and I diluted and then drank my Camelback. This was enough of a lift, but Brad, a keen student of psychology, also pointed out that the negative feelings I was experiencing were part of the natural way of things, the body was running down at the end of the day per the normal timetable of life, and that I would perk up once the night fell. And I did.

The rest of the race was a moving dream. I have only snatches of it in my memory. Jogging along the side of a valley on a cinder trail listening to the deafening soundtrack of a party blaring out from the black below me. Battling through fog, unable to see more than a few feet at a time, with my headlamp merely reflected back to me. Reaching La Turbie just above Monaco and seeing the sea for the first time since I had left the coast a couple of days previously. On my last legs, and having to make one last climb before the final aid station. Seeing Brad again at the aid station and surprising everyone by nearly beating him to the finish, having floated down the last descent as if on a cloud of joy. He was driving. Grabbing the hands of my two eldest kids as I sprinted across the line. Immersing myself in the sea, clutching a baguette filled with ham, cheese and mayonnaise, in one hand, and a can of lager in the other, as the party on the beach continued in celebration of this glorious adventure!

Almost 30% of the entrants did not finish the Cro in 2010, but this was not out of the ordinary. I heard some complain to Pietro, the main organiser, that it was too difficult. His reply was that it was never billed as easy. If it were, then a finish would not be an achievement. The race was something to be celebrated, something to savour, something robust and weighty and prized. The race was tough because the terrain was tough, a product of millions of years of vicious winters and baking hot summers, creating stresses for the rocks, shaped into mountains. I felt that in the same way I was being shaped into something else. I was harder, tougher, both in body and in mind. As I cooled my legs in the sea, I hoped that somehow this would imprint on and inspire my kids, not only in sport but in life.

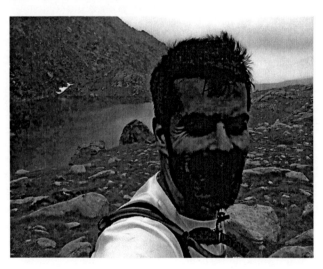

Somewhere on the Cro Magnon 2010 - Photo by Ben Rolfe

4 April 2011, Somewhere In The Sahara Desert

"Oh my God, I'm going to die!" I thought to myself as I saw the ground rushing up to meet me.

"I've done all this bloody training, preparation, travelled for the last 48 hours, and here I am within spitting distance of the campsite, and I'm going to break my neck falling off the bloody truck."

I was in the best shape of my life, having trained for eight months to take part in the Marathon Des Sables, a seven day Ultra Marathon across the Sahara Desert, billed by the organisers as the "Toughest Footrace on Earth".

I had returned to real life after the euphoria of the finish of the Cro Magnon. A few weeks after that, I had had a recurrence of my skin issue, with a freckle removed from just below my left arm pit, fortunately excising the dubious cells in one fell swoop. The phone call from the doctor with the results of the biopsy had been no easier to receive, however.

At work, the long hours of graft had been paying off, but I had decided that I wanted more autonomy and transparency on the profits in the longer term. A few weeks before I arrived in the desert I had quit the company I had worked so hard to help build over the previous eight years. It was like a weight was lifted from my shoulders.

Whilst I was in great physical shape, I had been in terrible mental shape. The only way I was keeping it together was to distract myself with every single race I could find. In less than a year, I had run the San Francisco marathon, Nice to Cannes Marathon, Gorbio trail marathon, Trail des Alpes Maritimes ultra marathon, an endurance triathlon (similar to a half Ironman), and the London Ultra 50km/30 mile race.

During that time I had received an invite from the organisers of the Marathon Des Sables to apply to their race, and I was rewarded with a place for April 2011. This was a fabled race, one on my bucket list, and had a three year waiting list. I had no idea how I had gotten so lucky. (Apparently I had registered on some database somewhere and my number came up!)

As a result, I had bitten the bullet, paid the entry [7]and started to accumulate kit. Two years after the seed of an idea had been sewn by my friend (who had not even made the start line of the Neander Trail), I had flown out with the French contingent from Paris to the Marathon Des Sables.

I had trained both in and out the gym for the previous couple of months with enough layers to embarrass the Michelin Man to try and assimilate my body to temperatures of more than 50 degrees Centigrade (122 Fahrenheit) that I was expecting to encounter.

I was between jobs and had time on my hands to take the kids to school and help with household chores (how I had ever fitted a job in as well was a mystery).

"Dad! What are you wearing?"

"I'm going for a run after dropping you off."

"But Daaaaaad! You look like you're in the Foreign Legion. So embarrassing!! Make sure you stand away from me."

"Come over here and give me a cuddle darling."

"NO WAY! GO AWAY!"

For the final couple of weeks before the race I enjoyed embarrassing the kids on the school run; I would take them on the Monaco bus from home to school before going for a training run myself. I was using my runs like a dress rehearsal for the race, in full desert kit with pack, cap, and gaiters. More than once I received a comment that I looked like a Foreign Legionnaire.

As we proceeded to the start, I prepared myself for imminent crushing between desert floor and Moroccan

---

[7] Somewhere in the region of €2000 in 2011. This included flights, hotel accommodation and food outside of the race itself, and huge medical and backup support.

Army Truck. Having arrived in Ouarzazate, I was crammed into the back of a Moroccan army flat bed truck with thirty other participants and volunteers plus all their kit bags, travelling the last kilometre or so to the first campsite. The campsite was a horseshoe of about 80 Berber tents, each one little more than a rug on a pole with sides open to the elements, eight to a tent. We would then go through a couple of days of initial checks before setting off on our seven day adventure.

I had been standing right on the edge of the truck, the weight of the other people pushing me out as we lurched over the uneven desert floor, more rocks than sand. To steady myself, I was holding an arched bar which would normally support a tarpaulin to keep off the scorching desert sun. The sun was the least of my worries however, as the bar came away in my hands, and both bar and I were pitched over the edge. Just as my feet lost contact with the chipped metal bed of the truck, the momentum shifted and the truck lurched violently in the opposite direction; the metal flew up, gathering me up as it went, and I was thrown on top of my pack and two other (quite annoyed) runners.

My pulse high and my palms sweaty, I dismounted a short time later, resisting the temptation to emulate the Pope and kiss the ground in thanks for my safe delivery. I looked for my pre-arranged tent-mates whom I had met on the blogosphere.

As part of my preparation for the race I had performed hundreds if not thousands of Google searches hungry for any and all information about training methods, kit preparation, how hot it was really going to be, and what to do if bitten by a camel spider (thankfully the seal on my venom pump remains, at the time of writing, unbroken). I came across a few blogs with race reports which had proven to be interesting and educational. As part of the natural progression of these things, I "met" a chap, Richard, who had been due to run the MdS with his wife, Liz, and their friends Anthony and Greg.

I had met up with Greg whilst in London for a sort of "tent mate" interview, and we had arranged to share a tent together. Greg already had an MdS finisher's medal, and knew the ins and outs of finding a tent, geographic location in the camp, and so on. With over a hundred competitor tents pitched in a horseshoe layout, it was important to be as near to the finish as possible to reduce the amount of extra agony piled on by walking to one's tent after a long, hot day trudging through sand or climbing over slate mountains.

Richard, sadly, was badly injured in a trail race the previous year, and was suffering an *annus horribilis* with a series of surgeries to rebuild the top of his femur and hip. We have still only met in the virtual world!

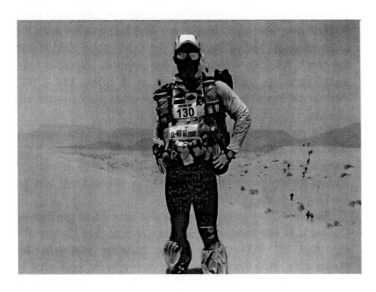

Sand - Photo by Ben Rolfe

6 April 2011, Day One, Bivouac 2

I had made it.

The first stage of the Marathon Des Sables was under my belt. I was, however, in a very bad way. As sods law dictated, I was injured. I had spent the last ten kilometres of the thirty–something kilometre "dune stage" trudging across the flat desert plane carrying my backpack in front of me, like a baby in my arms.

The Marathon Des Sables is a race totalling six marathons (250km/104 miles) in six stages of varying lengths. The race takes place in the Northern Sahara desert in Southern Morocco, and other than a rough Berber tent with open sides, and one and a half litres of water provided by the organisers every ten kilometres, the race is entirely self-sufficient. In practise, that meant carrying enough food to last for seven days, sleeping bag, toilet roll (with the cardboard removed, to save weight), extra clothes, and a whole raft of safety and scary medical gear such as the anti-venom pump. On top of all that, the organisers thoughtfully included a very heavy emergency flare. This had been compulsory equipment since the 1994 edition when the Italian policeman and former Olympic athlete, Mauro Prosperi, had wandered off course in a sandstorm and been lost in the desert for ten days, surviving only through drinking his own urine and bat's blood. Most of the competitors, myself included, would have probably gone down the piss and blood route as well, rather than fire the disqualification rocket.

The organisers took safety very seriously; the medical infrastructure included an army of race volunteers, a multitude of medical staff, two helicopters, and an airplane. Whilst there were inherent dangers, noone had died in the race since 2007. That year, very sadly, Bernard Jule, died in his sleep after crossing the finish line of the "long day", a double marathon. He was by all accounts a terrific athlete, was at the sharp end of the rankings, and had passed the stringent medical tests just to gain entry to the event. He woke to welcome some of his slower tent mates home at 3.30am, and was found dead of a heart attack at 6.30am. There was nothing that a huge army of medics could have done. All the competitors were aware that, despite the massive safety net, there were always very grave risks.

The course varied from year to year, although was broadly run along the same lines. Day One was the "Dune Stage", Day Four was the "Long Day" which would spill over into Day Five, and Day Six always the "Marathon Day", a full marathon despite having already travelled the best part of 200km in the previous week. Each stage was timed, and the cut off was strictly enforced with two camels, nicknamed Charles and Camilla, who lurched along behind the participants. If you were overtaken by the Royal couple, you would be withdrawn from the race. A local version of the sweeper bus.

I had no idea what to expect before I started, our camp was in a relatively flat area of the desert and conserving my energy I did not stray too far from the bivouac. The night before the start, when the two MdS veterans in my tent spoke calmly about mini Alps, the virgins (myself included), were sceptical. However, the organisers warned us that on occasion they would double our ration of water as the course was about to become inaccessible. That ration would obviously have to last for twenty kilometres rather than the usual ten.

I had been well schooled in the art of desert races by Mad Dog Mike, a veteran of multi stage ultras although never the MdS, and had also done a lot of research on the internet. I had resolved to take every drop of water as soon as it was offered by the organisers. Later on down the line – that day, or even later in the week, dehydration could be the difference between finishing and firing that flare.

In practise, this meant putting one and a half litres of water in my bottles, plus the same again as a dead weight on the pouch I carried on my chest. In training, this had not been too much of an issue, but as I was to find out, nothing can prepare you for the Sahara desert.

Day One.

The sand dunes were as high as tower blocks. An interminable section of dune after dune after dune, in searing heat with no cloud or shade. Going up was like trudging through porridge, each foot sinking several inches into the soft, fine sand. Coming down was more fun, as I could speed up a bit, but each strength sapping step took its toll on my mental strength too. Meanwhile, the water in my front pouch hanging from my shoulder straps, bounced around on my stomach like a medicine ball. Each bounce was painless in isolation, but the accumulated pounding over the first few hours of the race had given me severe deep muscle bruising and burst blood vessels.

I sat there in the finishing area, just coming up to the hottest part of the day, and sipped my complementary cup of sweetened Sultan herbal tea – nectar from heaven at the end of every stage – and debated on whether I could carry on the race. I wasn't sure what I was going to do ; there was only so far sheer determination could take me.

I grabbed that evening's ration of water – one and a half litres to last me until the start of the next day's stage - and tried to juggle my pack and the water bottles back to my tent.

Greg was already in the tent, laid out on the rug propped up on his pack, and ready to welcome me with a warm smile. He and I had become firm friends in the run up to the MdS. Over the course of the race, our tent was to form a bond that would last a lifetime.

I chatted with Greg about my injury, made myself some rehydrated spaghetti bolognaise, and took a couple of Nurofen. Greg was very supportive, and suggested I visit the Doc Trotters medical tent. Doc Trotters was the nickname given to the medical staff because over the course of the week 90% of the injuries were foot related, mainly infected blisters, as well as dehydration and the occasional broken bone.

I waited my turn. This was yet another part of the MdS experience, washing and disinfecting one's feet before entering the queue and then sitting on director's chairs in two rows facing each other, attempting to make conversation in the searing heat. When a stretcher came free, the medical orderly assigned to me seemed surprised to be dealing with something other than feet. He turned his attention to my visibly swollen shoulder. It was almost as if I was growing another head, the swelling was so bad. After a short period of poking and prodding, accompanied by sharp intakes of breath and occasional whelps (from me) he declared that in order for it to get better, I should withdraw from the race.

7 April 2011, Day Two

We waited nervously whilst any exposed skin was sandblasted. I was absolutely freezing despite being in the middle of the Sahara Desert. Trying to shelter from the wind and stay warm, we watched while they put a third IV drip into a chap from the neighbouring tent. He was lying prone, still in his sleeping bag, and the Berbers had removed his tent from above his head.

This wasn't entirely out of the ordinary. The team of Berbers that accompanied the MdS caravan drove a phalanx of army trucks. Every day they had to disassemble the tents, pack them in the trucks, drive to the site of the next bivouac and then set up the new camp, all before the first runners of the day finished their stage. We very quickly became accustomed to being woken by the Berber warbling, and the tents disappearing before we had even emerged from our sleeping bags.

I had awoken more tired than when I went to bed the night before. The tent had collapsed several times in the night due to the wind, and each time my head popped out of the sleeping bag it was like being stuck in a wind tunnel with someone throwing in handfuls of sand. We had therefore stayed in our sleeping bags whilst we watched the drama a few metres away. Unfortunately the chap on the receiving end of his third IV bag of saline solution couldn't actually get out of his.

It turned out that he was an Aussie, and he was going for highest place Aussie overall in the Marathon Des Sables. He had come into the race highly trained, but on the back end of a stomach bug, and was dehydrated before the first day. He had exacerbated this by not taking the extra water offered (the extra water which nearly knocked me permanently out of the race by bruising my shoulder so severely I finished the previous day's stage holding my pack like a baby). He had also been guilty of one of Mad Dog Mike's cardinal sins – going out too quickly. This was key to Mad Dog's doctrine, and for a stage race this meant not only pacing each stage, but pacing over the whole event. It was important to have negative splits every day and over the week – meaning that the first half should be slower than the second half.

After the third IV, the Aussie was able to sit up, but his race was over. He was bundled into a four wheel drive and taken away. No long term damage done, except to his pride. There had been several other withdrawals that day – one broken leg and one heart attack. Both went on to make full recoveries. One female competitor had not made the cut off, but would be given another chance to make up the time today. Every competitor had to finish each stage within a certain time marked by Charles and Camilla the Sultan Tea camels. Day One had taken me almost five and a half hours to do 33km, so I was no longer worried that Charles and Camilla would finish before me; my immediate worry was whether I would be able to carry my pack on my shoulders for the next 217 kilometres of desert.

Greg had finished Stage One ahead of the rest of us, and I was not far behind despite my injury. Anthony, the eye doctor, was third, with James, Clint, Liz, and Scott close on our heels. We were all chuffed to have got the first stage under our belts, but a few of us weren't exactly unscathed. Clint's feet were already starting to become problematic with blisters, James had a dead leg (possibly some sort of blood flow problem due to tight muscles, but it meant he did not have full mobility or control), Liz was finding it tough going because her training schedule had been very interrupted with her husband Richard's surgeries and looking after four kids and an invalid husband. But overall we were still in pretty good spirits.

Greg did a great job wrapping up my shoulder. He had purchased a Berber scarf from one of the initial bivouac merchants, and was using it as a pillow. He formed some sort of padding under my pack strap to prevent further bruising, and with some judicial rearrangement of the strap mechanism, I found I was able to support my pack without too much pain or strain. I looked like some sort of cross between a lycra clad Power Ranger, a Foreign Legionnaire, and a desert nomad. Still, looking bizarre would be the least of my worries after seven days and 250km without changing my clothes.

8 April 2011, Day Four, Part One. "Pain is temporary, memories last forever."

It was dark, I was on my last legs, and I was repeating this mantra to myself to keep me going through quite possibly the darkest hour I had ever felt at any point in my life. My body was telling my brain to just stop, just give up. I had been on my feet for thirteen straight hours, and I wasn't in truly great shape when I got up that morning. I felt in my bones now why The Marathon Des Sables is billed as the "Toughest Footrace on Earth". My whole body concurred.

Any veteran of the MdS stated that it was all about the Long Day; pacing was the key. The Long Day was 82km / 52 miles– a double marathon – through the desert with terrain which included sand up to my knees, and mountains covered in loose rocks, like Alps, to cross. Each competitor had already covered the first three stages, a 32km Dune Day, and a couple of 37km days with mixed terrain. Despite my shoulder injury I had ignored Doc Trotter's advice, and I was doing okay. The previous two nights had been tough with sandstorms whipping through the camp. I had woken up with a cold sore the size of a house, and feeling like I needn't have bothered going to sleep.

When the organisers said "Long Day", they meant it. Each competitor would have 36 hours to complete the distance. There were Berber Tents positioned along the course at Checkpoints and runners could bed down for a few hours if they needed to. Greg and I planned to push on through – whilst not at the very sharp end of the rankings, we were both within a shout of a top 15% finish. Plus, the sooner we finished, the longer we could rest, hopefully for the whole of the next day.

The trouble was, from about eleven hours in, I had hit my breaking point. The usual fatigue I experienced at nightfall never seemed to lift. Greg had lent me his trail sticks as I was noticeably slowing. We had started that day well, with a very disciplined ratio of 9:1, which is nine minutes jogging, one minute walking, a technique instilled in me from the very beginning of my ultra running career by Mad Dog Mike. We walked through the porridge-like sand (running through it was not an option) and we walked through the heat of the day (up to 50 degrees centigrade), with cracked lips and dry mouths, aghast when the leading Moroccan runners overtook us.

This was awe inspiring. The Moroccan guys ran like gazelles over anything the desert threw at them. The organisers realised that the top 50 runners would be significantly quicker than the majority of the field, and therefore gave everyone else a three hour headstart. Greg and I had managed to cover a significant distance before the first of the top 50 overtook us, just coming into the heat of the day. We crossed a dried lakebed – the sun baking us where we walked, and dodged various obstacles such as wild camels, goats, and a chap on a scooter. Those Honda 90's get everywhere, even the middle of the Sahara desert!

After trudging through the heat, it came as a relief when the sun began to wane. We were able to trot a little again. We stopped at the fourth checkpoint of the day, and whilst my gaiters were suffering a little, I patched them with a bit of gaffer tape, and changed my socks (the first and only change of clothes I allowed myself the whole week). Our aim was to get to the dunes by dusk. We had been warned that the local Berber kids found it amusing to move the trail markers. For the night sections, the markers glowed in the dark, and this included some dunes. If one of the markers was taken by local miscreants, it was not uncommon for people with little or no navigational experience to be found wandering around in circles in the dunes when the sun came up the next day. Having done our homework the night before, we identified the dunes as the most critical stage, and kept up a steady tempo through the huge lumps of sand, emerging just as the sun disappeared.

We arrived at the next checkpoint, lit our glow sticks and headlamps, and set off immediately. Before long we could see the laser in the sky – like a huge green light sabre upright in the clear desert night, denoting where camp was. It was a moment of elation which was to be steadily eroded – the sky was so clear and uncluttered by western light pollution, that the laser could be seen up to 25km in advance, a long way in the desert in the dark. Greg and I used a motivational technique I called fishing, to pass the time.

It was literally to "fish" people in – cast an imaginary rod, sink the hook into a person a few hundred metres ahead, jogging for a bit to catch them up, and then walking together for a spell, chatting, to cheer us all up. We would then repeat the procedure, using the technique to reel in the next person. We stopped briefly to admire a skull picked clean by vultures and bleached by the sun, and made our way steadily forward.

About 10km from the finish of the Long Day, I was finished. The heat, dehydration, hunger and fatigue had taken its toll. Greg had brought a pair of trekking poles which he claimed helped him as it kept everything moving, and helped take the weight a little from the legs. We were taking it in turns to use them and repeating the mantra "Pain is temporary, memories last forever." This had been told to me by a very good friend named Stuey O'Grady – a professional cyclist and one of the toughest sportsmen I had ever encountered, who rode in more Tour de Frances than anyone else ever. He claimed to use this mantra in the dark moments, pouring rain or snow, freezing cold, cycling over cobbles, when he felt he couldn't continue.

My headlamp illuminated a black scorpion scuttling across the dirt in front of me. Under normal circumstances, I would have flinched and shied away, but I was past caring; it was enough of an effort to put one foot in front of another. Greg managed to break into a trot and I joined him, briefly, before spluttering to an arthritic shuffle, shoes kicking up dust as they dragged along at the end of my legs. We skirted a small dune – the sand firmer at the bottom, all the while keeping the green laser in sight. As we crested the horizon, the desert floor below us was lit up by the lights of the finish line and the camp. We were overwhelmed. And overjoyed?

It was as if all the fatigue, hunger, thirst and sheer pain had been removed by a magic wand, and we ran full tilt to the finish line to be hugged by the beige clad volunteers, to the soundtrack of the deafening diesel generators that were keeping the laser and floodlights running. It had taken us just over thirteen hours to cover that day's stage, 23 hours ahead of the last competitor that crossed the line.

We grabbed our water ration for the night, and waddled back to the tent. The other tents were almost empty, just the odd sleeping back dotted here and there lying on the Berber rugs, like human sized cocoons, concealing bodies exhausted from the cumulative exertions of the week. We found our tent, and attended to our "admin" – in my case this meant finding something solid to eat.

I had spent months preparing for the MdS, sourcing and trying out various freeze dried foods, including generic looking powder that with a little added water and some heat became high carb sludge. I had re-packed these with a vacuum sealer saving a kilo of weight in the process, and then parcelled everything up into seven ration parcels. The rules stated that each competitor should have a minimum of 2000 calories per day – about the minimum recommended daily intake for a human adult in order to survive. I had about 2500 per day – consisting of a freeze dried porridge, tea bag and Berocca vitamin for breakfast, Peanut M&M's, raisins and fried peanuts as a homemade trail mix for snacks on the go, a couple of 9Bars or Go Bars to augment the trail mix. For my evening meal I had a variety of freeze dried lasagne or spaghetti bolognaise followed by a freeze dried pudding. I estimated that I used more than 13000 calories during the long run day, so at the very least I would be losing a bit of weight! I had decided not to take any crockery or stove, as I could chop the bottom off one of the water bottles I was given my ration in, and use that as a cup. Instead of a stove, I was a dab hand at semi burying my sludge like concoctions in the sand and letting it be heated – through the clear plastic – by the sun.

Greg and I had finished the long day at around 10.30pm at night – the sun was long gone, and the desert temperature was dropping fast. During the night it could get down to just above freezing, and I was cold, tired and needed to eat having only eaten a bar and some trail mix during the day. I mixed up my sludge and forced down a couple of spoonfuls without waiting for the pasta to soften from the consistency of broken chicken bones. I wretched, and crawled into my sleeping bag. Greg had thrown his stove out the first day and was following my lead, but seemed to be enjoying his evening meal more than I was. I forced down another couple of spoonfuls and then collapsed into a heap in my sleeping bag.

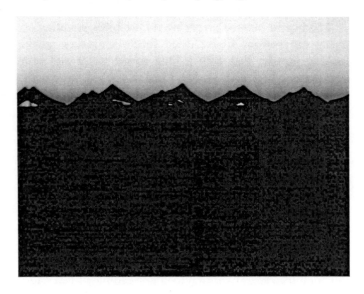

Well ventilated tents - Photo by Ben Rolfe

9 April 2011, Day Four, Part Two

Eyes caked in gunk, dried salt falling off me in flakes, I looked around, completely disoriented. My whole body ached, and I was starving, but for a few seconds I was like a newborn with absolutely no idea of where I was. The night was clear and there was enough ambient light to see my immediate surroundings – and it all came back to me. The filthy carpet on the floor, the Berber tent made from a black rug draped over a couple of poles, and the cool desert air. The tent housed only me, Greg and another body wrapped up in a sleeping bag, unconscious. I pressed the light on my watch; it was 3.30am, and only three out of the seven of us from the tent had so far made it back on the "Long Day" – the double marathon day, of the Marathon Des Sables. I got up to go for a pee, ease some of the stiffness from my aching body, and finish off the rehydrated pasta I hadn't eaten the night before. As I hobbled arthritically, painfully, towards the outer limits of the camp, I could see that three out of eight to a tent was a decent return so far. A lot of the tents had single people in, and some remained completely empty. The pain of walking across the sharp flinty rocks in my slippers, little more than a couple of socks on the soles of my feet, dissipated with a certain rush of pride. Greg and I had been in for five hours, and we were still very much at the sharp end of the pack. As I relieved myself by the light of the stars, I looked across the desert at the finish line of Stage Four, the entrance to the horseshoe shaped camp, and I could see a broken line of headlamps as competitors made their way to the finish. Replete, relieved, and very satisfied, I hobbled back to the tent and oblivion once again.

Later, the distant sound of people talking woke me. My Pavlovian reaction was to immediately get up and start dressing and packing for that day's stage. The empty tent served to remind me that this was day two of the "Long

Day". Actually there was no hurry to do anything. During the night, Anthony, Scott and James had come in, and we were now only missing Clint and Liz. It was emotional seeing the others, and even though it was only 7.30am they blinked themselves awake and were happy to chat and discuss the adventures of the day.

"Did you see the skull?"

"Yeah! What do you think it was?"

"A goat?"

"Baby camel?"

"Who knows but one of the other blokes picked it up and was taking photos with it."

"He picked it up? Jesus! I hope he washed his hands."

After our experiences watching the Aussie competitor being put on multiple drips and sent home on Day One, we had all become very wary of illness and disease. We had been warned to steer clear of any water offered by anyone along the way or from local wells. We mulled over our experiences, and shouted greetings at any feet we recognised passing by our tent, as people made their way back to their lodgings.

I spent the whole day resting, queuing for the emails tent to write the precious one email per day I was allowed, watching the finishers, and eating anything and everything I could get my hands on. The last person reached our tent at 11am – a great achievement particularly as Clint's feet had no skin on the soles at all; they resembled a raw, skinned, chicken underneath. At this, there wasn't a dry eye in our tent.

A great tradition of the Marathon Des Sables is the camaraderie throughout the whole camp, and this is demonstrated in full when the leaders of the race come out and applaud the last person to complete the "Long Day". 2011 was no different, and towards the end of the afternoon a growing stream of people were passing the tent to join the crowd gathering to cheer in the last of the runners.

I stood shoulder to shoulder with Mohamad Ahansal, something of an MdS legend (having won it three times), and the current leader of the race, as we watched the last stragglers of the race hobbling across the last few kilometres. They were making achingly slow progress, as small as Lego figures on the horizon, and probably with about the same range of mobility. They were just ahead of the camels with their characteristic lurching from side to side accompanied by the blue clad Berber handlers, the desert sweeper bus. There was a desperate game of cat and mouse being played out in slow motion in front of our eyes, the three runners pulling ahead a few metres, slowing down, Charles and Camilla almost catching them, until they scurried ahead again. We waited at the finish, aching bodies draped on tea chests or slumped on the floor, willing the last runners home. 66 people had dropped out that day alone, most due to dehydration and fatigue, but this little gaggle of three were determined to finish. A few of their tent mates and team members walked out to meet them, and give them as much of a boost as possible. Everyone in the crowd was cheering, although no one wanted to walk further than was strictly necessary as the next day we still had a sandy, windy and hilly marathon to complete. Our support was spiritual and verbal.

The figures gradually neared, not so much Lego pieces as Action Men sized now. It was clear they were struggling but with another big cheer and a clap from the crowd they broke into a very slow trot. The relief throughout the camp was palpable. I looked around and several of the dirty faces were tear stained, as every single competitor felt empathy with the finishers – Mohamad included. The pain and relief on the faces of those last couple of runners was clear for all to see, and leaving them to their private thoughts, I turned and went back to my tent to rehydrate some supper and bed down for the night.

10 April 2011, Day Six, Marathon Stage, Sahara Pavement Pizza

"Ca va?" I asked.

The Marathon des Sables was an event organised by the French, and the vast majority of the volunteers and the greatest proportion of participants were French. Having lived in France for eight years, I had picked up a little bit of the language – enough to have a trail chat anyway.

"Are you ok mate?" I tried a different tack, as I had not received a response to my initial enquiry. The object of my small talk was bent over, in that peculiar but extremely familiar pose of the extremely uncomfortable. His legs were slightly apart, a small patch of damp earth and rock between his battered trainers. The wind was whipping up the dust, drying out the product of his heaving body almost before it had hit the ground. The race was truly taking its toll.

"Feel much better now" He croaked, wearily straightening himself up like an old man, and licking the white flecks of dry salt and saliva from around his mouth.

"Keep your head up matey, not long to go now." I waved cheerily as I worked my way up to a slow trot. It was getting that way; almost like a heavy goods truck or ocean liner, it took a little while to build up momentum from standstill. I looked at my Garmin – only another 10km to go for the day, and effectively the race would be all but over, with just the liaison stage of 17km the following day before a shower, proper food, another shower, and a bed. With a mattress! It was like being drunk I was so euphoric.

My air mattress had popped the previous day, and I had spent the night sleeping on jagged rocks using my punctured air bed as an ineffective pillow. I had run / walked / climbed / crawled / shuffled for the best part of 225km in six days, and I was three quarters of the way through the marathon (42.2km) stage of the race, with the promise of the Paris Philharmonic Orchestra in camp that evening.

The day had started well. The previous evening we had all been given a soda and a new number, the only clean thing I had on my person. Everything else was coated in layers of dust, blood, snot and iodine, which seemed to be the main causes of grime in the camp, in addition to pus. Greg and I had discussed tactics that day, having run the majority of the race in tandem. Greg was very keen to break 5 hours for the marathon stage. I wanted to pace myself, just like Mad Dog had taught me. I started the stage as I had the others with nine minutes jogging, one minute walking. Walk the deep sand. Walk uphill, sprint downhill. It had served me well, and I was determined not to break strategy at this juncture. Greg and I followed procedure for the first half, and then he pulled away from me. We had agreed to run the marathon per our own plan rather than as a pair. A marathon seemed easy in comparison to everything we had already been through, and besides, for me to set off too quickly would have only added to the time outside camp later on.

It was clear that the race was taking its toll, as I passed the leading woman pretty early on. She was broken and on the verge of pulling out. People were limping, lying down at checkpoints, generally looking haunted as I passed them. It was like the retreat from Stalingrad, with the 1000 yard stare and hollow cheeks demonstrating the toughness of the race.

My gaiters were shredded. I had had them made from parachute material and stitched to my trainers to stop the sand from getting into my shoes. I had patched them as much as I could with gaffer tape. My trainers weren't unscathed either. They were missing great big chunks from both heels. The heat had literally melted the glue and running downhill had ripped the heels off. I had used dental floss (stronger than cotton and packed in preparation) to sew up my t-shirt and shorts in various places. I had no alternatives; patch up and go was the only viable strategy.

In complete contrast to some of the other competitors and my dishevelled appearance, I was having an absolute ball.

As I ran into one checkpoint, I used the filtering railings as a piece of gymnastics equipment, putting my hands on the top – one on each railing, and pushing down to lift my feet off the ground. When asked by the medical staff in attendance whether I was ok, I shouted "IMPECCABLE" at them, and laughed. A cameraman saw me and swung round to capture my mood. I took a few seconds to fill my water bottles, and then ran out of the Checkpoint area being chased by the cameraman, filming my euphoria! Sadly I was never able to locate the film, perhaps the cameraman had not had time to switch on his machine as I was moving so fast!

The complete aridity and barrenness of the desert was giving way to tiny signs of civilization. Primitive irrigation channels were visible, and whilst we did not pass through any settlements, there were definitely more people about, mainly children asking for food and sweets. I thought to myself as I passed the umpteenth gaggle of young kids with upturned palms and mischievous smiles, that they were barking up the wrong tree. I had carefully weighed and measured every single calorie for the whole week, and even repacked a lot of the food to cut down weight further, and I had nothing to spare. I had noticeably slimmed down during the race. Maybe another competitor would be happy to offload a few M&Ms to the hungry locals.

I crossed the line into the last bivouac of the race, and I was absolutely overcome with emotion, finishing the marathon stage in about 5 hours and 20 minutes, not a bad marathon time considering there had been quite a bit of altitude to negotiate, in addition to the heat and terrain. Effectively, the race for me was over. All that remained was the short liaison stage in the morning which I was confident I could run in less than two hours. The tears would not stop coming, as I had the last cup of complimentary Sultan tea. Nectar.

I cried all the way back to my tent, whilst I made myself a small meal, when I had emailed my wife, and I was in absolute floods of tears when the Paris Orchestra (flown in to entertain the sponsors and VIPs) played their music, done up in black tie, in a shallow natural amphitheatre, about 100 metres from the tents.

Later that evening I got up to relieve myself, putting on what was left of my slippers. I hobbled a few yards from the tents, ground ahead of me lit only by my headlamp, and had a pee facing away from the camp. Earlier in the week, I had been fastidious about leaving the cordon, about 100 metres from the outer ring of tents, and peeing behind a dune or a shrub. Not so on the last night. My feet were tender, made all the more so by the thin covering of complementary hotel slippers, not in great shape themselves. The ground underfoot was littered with jagged bits of slate, sharp and uncomfortable.

I could hear sharp intakes of breath not far from me.

"Ouch. Ooof. Flip."

Someone was not having a great time of it. I turned without thinking about it, highlighting with my headlamp a 30 something year old woman who had been in a neighbouring tent all week. It was clear she was a multi-ultra finisher, very experienced and probably used to being on the podium a lot of the time, the way she spoke. The desert was a great leveller. Every step she took was an effort, the pain written on her dirty and salt encrusted face.

"Oh fuck it." She was only about two metres from the tents when she dropped her tights and peed on the spot. Enough was enough! I turned away, smiling into the distance.

11 April 2011, Day Seven, Liaison Stage

My pack was flapping around on my back not so much a rucksack as a loose flap of cloth, and I was able to get quite a pace up as the sand gave way to tarmac underfoot. I was playing the fishing game again, perfected on numerous runs, not least of which crossing the Sahara Desert. There were not so many runners in front of me as I sprinted onto the tarmac – I was in the top 10% for the day, and I was putting in a reasonable time. The fatigue accumulated through the race was lifting. That morning I could barely drag myself out of my sleeping bag. My whole body was fit only for the knacker's yard, with dehydration and lack of sleep exacerbating an already critical situation. Temperatures had hit more than 50 degrees Centigrade daily, water was strictly rationed. We had had several sandstorms during the week, at night, making sleep a virtual impossibility. Not to mention a punctured air bed which for the past two nights had been about as welcome and useful as a discarded chocolate wrapper.

I felt every centimetre of those 250km. In six days. Across the Sahara Bloody Desert!

Greg and I had started the last stage together, but within a few hundred metres he pulled ahead, as my habit to start every stage extremely easy was fully ingrained. Most other people had also started very quickly, but within a few kilometres I had turned the tables, and the benefits of my pacing were paying dividends. I overtook Greg in Checkpoint One but did not stop. The scenery had been spectacular all week, and was now starting to get as familiar as a small town in the Sahara Desert can be. There were the usual Moonscapes of rocks, some soft sand and a jebel (mountain) or two to scale, but before long we were meandering through cultivated plots with vegetables and fruits growing. Little allotments had been carved out of the desert, with what little water there was available utilised sparingly to irrigate the agriculture. We had been instructed to take care of the land, and stick to the paths, and I was very careful to follow the advice as I understood how precious these fields were to the people surviving in this hostile environment.

I focussed on a group of runners in red as we started weaving our way through small dwellings, and as I hit tarmac I was able to open up and overtake them. It was a mere couple of km's to the finish and I ended the race like a 10km race – at a sprint - the sound of the commentator on the sound system booming from some unknown point ahead of me, pulling me.

I crossed the line at what seemed the speed of light, and was embraced by the race director Patrick Bauer before being presented with my medal, a moment forever etched onto my consciousness. Months of planning and years of training had led me to that point, an achievement I could only dream of a couple of years previously.

I managed to find someone from which to buy a Coke, and soaked in the atmosphere. A few VIPs, sponsors and supporters had flown to camp the previous day to experience what we, the runners, had gone through. They cheered, and looked awestruck as each competitor crossed the line to Patrick's embrace. A few years previously, crossing the finish line had been a mere pipe dream.

I am now a finisher of the Marathon des Sables, the "Toughest Footrace On Earth", I thought.

If I could do that, anything was possible.

17 April 2014, Lenval Hospital, Nice, France

The alarms screeched above my head, taking me back to the Sahara for a nano second. The electronic alarms were scarily close to the Berber singing as they dismantled base camp before dashing off to the next bivouac. If anything, I felt more exhausted than if I had been back in the desert, and wearily I turned over. I was greeted with a face full of soft, matronly buttock, thankfully encased in surgical scrubs. I peeled my face from the vinyl pillow, the faux leather pattern imprinted into my cheek, and moved back to give the nurse a little more room.

We had checked in earlier that day so that Alice could have a pump fitted. A few years ago, the medical profession developed a pump mechanism whereby a reservoir of fast acting insulin could be held near to the body and attached to the body with a tube via a catheter, and little bits of insulin could be released every three minutes. The pump could be programmed to release different amounts of insulin throughout the day according to that person's particular rhythm. Simultaneously, the pump enabled the wearer to plug in a certain amount of carbs into the interface on the pump, and the pump would release an appropriate amount of insulin, again allowing for different ratios of carbs to insulin depending on the time of day or night.

On Thursday 17th April, coincidentally Mrs R's 29th birthday, Alice and I checked in to Lenval in Nice - right on the sea front overlooking the Med. Mrs R came along for a bit before heading back home to deal with the other two kids who were still at school until the following evening, and it was my turn to sleep in hospital with Alice. I had joked that they should name a wing of the hospital after our family, we seemed to spend so much time there. There was the time Isabelle, my youngest daughter, bit off her tongue and had it reattached, when she was a year old. Another time one of the kids had appendicitis. I had visited the hospital a few times with various ailments including my post run collapse, and one fun time I had an anaphylactic shock after a delicious tuna steak. It felt like we spent a lot of time there, but in reality we are no different to any other family.

Whilst the pump negates the need for so many injections, there is still a lot to deal with. The cannula is not permanent - there is a small tube that has to be injected into the fat of the stomach every three days or so. The reason for this is that left in any longer and the risk of infection or blockage goes up. The pump insulin doses also need to be adjusted for the individual, and sometimes more than once a month depending on puberty, hormones, physical exercise and of course if Alice has a growth spurt. For this reason, the Diabetes clinic at Nice liked to keep children in for five days at a time. Mrs R and I had negotiated that down to three on the basis that we were actively taking an interest in Diabetes and helping Alice every step of the way. There were other kids in Lenval at the same time who had no accompanying parents at all.

On arrival at the hospital, Alice had the cannula inserted, appropriate doses of insulin dialled into the pump worked out by Dr Gastaud, and then we stayed in the hospital to get used to operating the pump, changing the cannula, and making sure that everything was working smoothly. We were shown to a room with a view – our home for a few days, which was set up for two child patients and two camp beds for parents. We occupied ourselves as best we could with books, games and videos, but every two hours a nurse would come by and perform a blood glucose check to make sure the doses were fine and Alice wasn't having a hypo or hyper. Every two hours, day and night.

The screech of alarms that woke me belonged to the boy in the neighbouring bed who had a gastrointestinal issue. The complication was that he was also a haemophiliac, but needed an operation to remove a small growth in his stomach. The screeching of alarms was due to his vital signs dropping below optimum or a blockage to the drip bags post the operation. Not only was I woken every two hours for Alice's blood sugar to be taken, but also when the boy in the bed next to me had issues. It was a long night, but in a sense there was a camaraderie between parents and patients. It made me all too aware that everyone is fighting their own battle, whether they are up front about it or not.

I awoke the next day at 8am as the new shift of nurses came in to check vitals, and to ensure we put the camp beds away before the various Dr's came to do their rounds. I felt like I had been on a three day bender. Alice was similarly tired, although in pretty good spirits as her friend, Lena, another Type One Diabetic from Monaco, had promised to come and visit that evening to break up the tedium. We had concocted a plan between us to escape for a while and meet her friend at a restaurant not far from the hospital, for dinner. We added several thousand forms to our already onerous paperwork sessions, and had another educational session on Ketones with the diabetic nurse that morning.

Ketones occur when a diabetic's blood sugar level is too high for too long, and they can be toxic. The treatment, if not too far advanced, is to administer more insulin. Because of the vagaries of the pump, blockages or mechanical issues can mean that although you think you are having the right dose of insulin, you may not have been having any insulin for a while, causing Ketones to build in your blood. We had read about Ketones before and had been educated about them at the Diabetes UK weekend, so were familiar with various treatments and doses.

The rest of our time in hospital was spent much the same way. I tried to remain limber with stretches and stationary exercises, the odd walk, read a few books, and played games with Alice. Our roommate bounced back and was discharged, and after three days we were released back into the wild with a couple of bags full of equipment and a series of follow-up appointments with various health professionals. Alice seemed pleased to not have to inject a minimum of four times a day, having cut that unpleasant aspect of her condition down to every three or four days. She also loved the attention from the kindly nurses who gifted her supplies of equipment bags and stickers for her pump. I was privately amazed but very pleased that she did not seem phased to have a pump permanently attached to her body, day and night.

I was a proud dad at how resilient and strong my sensitive little girl had become.

20 June 2014, Cro Magnon

As we hiked up the first of many steep climbs, affording spectacular views across the mountains, I shed layers, trying to stuff them in my backpack. Although I didn't really consider myself an elite athlete, I had had plenty of ultra running experience over the years, and had acquired quite a bit of kit that I was comfortable with. One unexpected side effect of the Cro, and my unusual challenge and slightly elevated profile as a result, was that one of the sponsors of the Cro had decided to provide me with a load of kit specifically designed for ultra trail running. A few weeks before I had received a large box of assorted t-shirts, shorts, over layers, and a waterproof jacket. I felt very privileged having previously bought kit in the January sales and made do. In that respect I felt very similar to Alice, the frisson of excitement at receiving Free Stuff that was Specifically For Me.

A monk rang a hand bell and smiled as we climbed past his seminary. We reached the summit and jogged through a ruined fort, a few wisps of clouds dissipating just above the tops of the walls. I took a moment to enjoy the view over the mountains and valleys as the sun came up, living the moment. This is what it was all about. The multitude of colours at sunrise, the verdant green of the summer mountain grass giving way to hard packed snow a few metres from where we were standing. I knew that the next few hours would test me to my absolute limit, having already covered an ultra marathon on the way to the start, but unless I reached my limits I would never know where they were.

I jogged slowly on the relatively flat cinder trail, happy to let others pass me in the early stages of the race. I knew, now more than ever, that I needed to keep everything in reserve. I kept an eye on my Garmin GPS as I still had various time limits to avoid disqualification, but I also needed to pay mind to my own body.

A river of snow crossed the trail, diagonally following the line of the hill from top left to bottom right. It had obviously built up over the winter and due to the unseasonably cold summer, it had not gone away. The snow was at head height blocking the whole trail apart from a thin passage cut into it to enable our passage. Not only had the organisers had to deal with a last minute route change, but the new course was not entirely without its challenges. This wasn't the first time I had encountered snow in my ultra running career, and I was glad that it wasn't the middle of the night and blowing a gale.

1 September 2012, 2am Lost in a snow storm

It had been some time since I had been able to feel my fingers or toes; all my extremities were just extra baggage I had to carry on my journey. I had started the race cold and wet, and was now freezing cold and freezing wet. I had long ago stopped shivering, which I knew was a bad sign – I was verging on hypothermic – but I was on the top of a mountain in the middle of the night, in a snowstorm, my feet sinking into a foot of fresh powder snow with every strength-sapping step, and I was completely lost.

I had been on my feet for seven hours or more, and had been using up critical stores of energy due to excessive stress and nerves, for several hours. I was participating in the Ultra Trail of Mont Blanc (UTMB) – a single stage 166km ultramarathon broadly following the Tour de Mont Blanc hiking path, with walkers taking somewhere in the region of 7-10 days to cover the distance. They would be rewarded with stunning views on their loop around the tallest mountain in Europe. Ten years previously, the first UTMB had taken place, and the race had very quickly taken on a life of its own, with 2500 racers in the UTMB, and many more undertaking one of the lesser races – the Courmayeur Champex Chamonix (CCC - 101km/63 miles), or Trace Des Duc de Savoie (TDS - 119km/74.5 miles) in the same region. Entries were prized for all three races, with the UTMB the pinnacle of every ultrarunner's bucket list. A complex points system of qualification had been devised, and even then each place was oversubscribed 3:1. I had been fortunate enough to qualify through the MdS and Cro, and was participating in the foremost ultramarathon in Europe.

I had arrived in Chamonix on 29th August on my own, knowing no one racing, and not having any support. It felt odd doing the race as an individual in the truest sense of the word, and the sense of loneliness was heightened by the check-in procedure as I queued for the registration and equipment checks, with large groups of chiselled runners, and families with kids milling around. My French, despite residing in the country for nine years, still wasn't that great, and after the tiniest amount of small talk with those around me I was very quickly left to my own thoughts.

I had time to reflect on my training, and the recent journey that had taken me there. Greg had given me the idea for the UTMB during the MdS as we whiled away the hours chatting during and after each day's stage. One of the first things I did on my return was to look up Greg's blog report on the UTMB. I had entered, only half expecting to get a place and had been rewarded with one, although I had been unsuccessful in my attempts to recruit an accompanying nutter. My last remaining "crew" had dropped out that very day, due to inclement weather on the way to Chamonix. I had just made it through the storm in time.

Eventually I reached the front of the queue, and it was my turn to get my equipment checked. I had spent an immense amount of time to gather the kit to fulfil the compulsory requirements and my own wants and needs, as well as fit it all into a small backpack and focus on being as light as possible. I was almost disappointed when the wizened old Chamois volunteer gave my rucksack – of which I was extremely proud, the most cursory of glances. I picked up all the other goodies – a rubbish bag, drop bag, dossard (race number), identity bracelet, and the all important participant t-shirt. I emerged from the marquee into freezing torrential sleety rain, punctuated with thunder and lightning. I made my way back to my hotel on the outskirts of Chamonix, had an early dinner, got an early night, and fell asleep praying for good weather.

I had not poured enough of a libation to the running Gods as my prayers had most definitely not been answered. I woke early the next morning to an SMS from the organisers to say that due to excessive snow, which was still falling, they were unsure whether there was actually going to be a race. It was considered to be too dangerous to the participants and volunteer marshals. They had actually shortened the CCC and cancelled the TdS as a result of bad weather.

I felt like the world had been taken away from me. I was utterly devastated. All that training, preparation, dedication, and the time away from the family was potentially going to go to waste. Not to mention all the pledges for donations I had received for charity which I would no longer be able to collect on. I looked out the window at Mont Blanc herself, and in complete contrast to the previous day, I was confronted with a snow covered mountain. Mont Blanc was living up to her name. Of course, the organisers only had our safety at heart, but it made the pill no less bitter to swallow. I prepared my stuff, and trudged down to breakfast, compulsively checking my phone for further SMS updates, much like an addict twitching for a fix.

After a meal and an abortive attempt at further rest, I heaved myself out of my bed and dressed for the race. Having had a brief walk around outside, and further carb loading, I decided that the best strategy was to wear the kit I was planning on wearing for the race, plus everything that I was planning on carrying in my pack for the peaks. This consisted of shorts, tights, t-shirt, thermal top, jacket and Gore Tex. I had thick mountain-biking gloves, running beanie, woollen beanie and waterproof over-trousers as well. Looking a bit like Mr Staypuft from Ghostbusters, I caught the bus to the centre of Chamonix, and gathered with the rest of the nervous crowds in the main marquee. The weather was dry but cold; ominously, the cloud level was just above our heads, affording no view of the freshly snow-covered Mont Blanc.

Hand written posters had proliferated after lunch around town, stating that the race would continue, although with a heavily adjusted route. The passes out of France and into Italy and Switzerland, to my mind part of the attraction of the race, were in some cases blocked by more than two metres of snow. It was impossible to consider the original tour of Mont Blanc, but the organisers were desperate to hold some sort of race, as cancellations and weather-related chaos had marred a couple of the more recent versions of the UTMB. The new route was essentially a lap of the Chamonix valley, with around 6000 metres of positive altitude change, and something approximating 100km/62.5 miles of distance. No mean feat, but not the original race that I had looked forward to, and trained many months for. I was disappointed, but remained focussed on the race, and at least pleased to have some sort of race for my trouble. In the mountains, there is always the chance that weather will disrupt the best laid plans.

Ironically, the weather in the valley cleared as we restlessly milled around in the square for the start: a carpet of manmade fibre in hues of reds, blues, blacks and white. The final plans for the race were relayed to us over the tannoy, and the excitement was building. I tried to converse with a few people, with mixed success, the race so high profile that the mix of nationalities was endless. In the end I focussed on the commentator, and looked around to see if the more professional looking veterans had their headlamps on or not.

The square was so packed with runners, it was like being penned in at the start of a big city marathon, and the mood matched. A few words from the commentator about the conditions, and then a very stirring theme song blared out from the P.A. system – it was so loud I actually had to move away from the speakers near me! We were off, and the anxiety over actually having to go home with no blisters or fatigue, were left behind.

The narrow streets of Chamonix were packed with crowds, such that it was almost impossible to run with any conviction. People were high fiving runners, kids aglow with excitement, and I burst out laughing. This is what I loved! I could have lifted my legs off the ground and still been carried along by the surging current of runners, but I was racing, and loving it. Whatever the mountains had to throw at me, I shouted to myself, Bring It On!

That euphoria wore off after about fifteen minutes.

It started to rain, and I was already freezing cold. This was supposed to be late August for goodness sake, and it was reminiscent of a winter's trail run! Not only did I have to contend with the weather, but we were on single track trail, and I lost count of the number of times I was stabbed in the foot, thigh, and crotch with trail poles. I was not amused, and as a result made it my aim to get past as many people as possible in order to avoid serious injury, and to keep warm.

The trail widened, we hiked up a road, the sun fell, and so did the rain. At least the incline was warming me up, although I was not getting to see any of the scenery I had hoped for, but the crowds were out including a local family who had set up an impromptu aid station outside their house stocked with soup and jelly babies. I thanked them profusely, declining the sustenance but drawing strength and humour from their good natured banter and enthusiasm. Despite the course change, the spirit of the UTMB lived on.

The rain continued to fall, torrentially, and the UTMB runners continued to hike uphill. It was nice chatting to a few fellow English speakers, a rarity amongst my many races in France and Italy, and I met some really interesting people. One chap, Bruce, I had hooked up with on Twitter before the race; he had DNF'd the previous year, and had a point to prove. We approached a checkpoint with a bonfire and he recalled stopping for a long time there the previous year to warm up, something that he had pinpointed as to the start of his decline to DNF. It was difficult to compare the checkpoints to previous years, given the new course, and all my homework had been left behind in the rubbish bins, but I made a point of not going near the bonfire and just moving out of the checkpoint after refilling my backpack with water, and hiking onwards and upwards.

Literally metres later, I was hiking through snow, and my night became exciting for all the wrong reasons.

The snow was settling on the cinder trail, and my feet were leaving tracks, only to be filled in within seconds as the snow continued to blanket the ground. My feet and hands were beyond cold; I had on every layer of clothing I had brought with me, including both hats and two pairs of gloves, but it was no use considering the amount of rain that had fallen and the soaking I had been forced to endure before going through the snow line. Soon after reaching the snow, I crested the hill, and the old route had been blocked off with plastic ribbon. I was with a group of two or three other runners and we searched in vain for the new route's turn off. The land was semi cultivated for livestock, and there were little wire fences criss-crossing the fields, but there was no visible marking for the new route.

Fighting a rising sense of unease, in the dark, at altitude, in a snow storm, and about a foot of snow on the ground, we looked around us, the light from our LED headlamps reflecting back from the massive snowflakes forming a curtain of snow, blocking all but the most immediate of surroundings. I was thankful for my previous night running experience, and I was able to draw on some inner reserve to stay calm, unlike my running companions who were muttering in foreign languages to each other, and themselves, eyes wide with rising panic. Whilst the course was merely hours old, I had had a good look at the map pinned up in the marquee, and I knew that the turn off was not too far from the old course turn off, heading in roughly the same direction. I was guessing, but I thought we had gone too far as we were heading back down the hill, and according to the course notes and map the next section should have been flat or a small incline.

I made an executive decision, not overly bothered whether my peloton was going to stay with me or not; I had to protect myself first and foremost, and they weren't being a great deal of help. I hurdled the fence and headed parallel on a course with the uphill on my left, and the downhill on my right, circumnavigating the hill. I hoped that I would at some point intersect with the narrow footpath that would lead me back onto the course. Despite the poor visibility, the contours were guiding me, although that did not prevent me from tripping over an electric fence. After face planting into several centimetres of fresh snow, I picked myself up and a few steps later fell through some thin ice into a small, freezing cold stream.

My feet and hands were numb. I drew small comfort from my two colleagues who had decided to pin their hopes on me, God help them. Suddenly, one of them yelled. I looked where he was gesturing and through a break in the weather I could see a couple of bobbing LED's in the distance. We were on the right track. A few seconds later, and I could make out some distinct footprints in the snow leading off to the right, and I changed course to follow them.

Almost immediately the headlamps in front disappeared as the weather closed back in, as the path had been cut with an avalanche of rocks some time before. Possibly a few hundred or thousand years before. The UTMB course had been marked with chalk and tape, so I could see that I had to make my way over this obstacle, but the boulders were man-sized, so it was not going to be a small undertaking. My running partners were reluctant to take the lead, so I launched myself up the first rock, thank goodness for all the upper body training that Mad Dog Mike had put me through, preparing this race. Hauling myself from rock to rock became a sort of dance; it was all about getting into a rhythm and dragging first my upper body and then legs from rock to rock, a bit like the way a caterpillar moves along the ground. The weather was gradually lifting, and whilst I was still numb from the cold, I could at least see a little better, although with the headlamp bouncing around and crossing beams with those behind me, it was easy to get disorientated. I lost my balance and out of the corner of my eye saw a rock to my right – the downhill side of me. I put out my hand to steady myself and realised too late it was a little scrubby bush, and my hand passed straight through it, followed by my arm and then my chest. Prostrate on the floor, my thighs resting on one rock, my waist on the bush and my head, shoulders and arms extended into the dark emptiness, I looked down.

A tunnel was forming around me and it was like I was moving backwards through it, although there was no light at either end. Of course, I had stopped moving, but the constant falling snow was highlighted in my headlamp's beam, and falling past my head, briefly into my field of vision, before continuing its journey to the valley below, wherever that might have been.

I dragged myself first into a sitting position, and then stood up, preferring not to dwell too much on what had just happened and what could have happened. I looked around, and my running partners were standing there staring at me in stunned silence. Many thanks, chaps.

A long time later, and I was back in the valley, still on course, and into an aid station. There was a party going on: people drinking beer, a band playing AC/DC next to a huge two metre high bonfire. I struggled with my gloves to fill up my Camelback and have some hot soup. It must have been 3.30am, but the party around the UTMB continued. Whatever had happened, and whatever was to come, this was what it was all about. 'Normal people' would be at home watching tv, or perhaps down the pub having a drink with their mates in the warm, dry and safe environments afforded them. We, the people participating in the UTMB, whether runner or supporter, were doing something different, daring, and learning something about ourselves in the process.

I staggered in to Chamonix around 3pm on the Saturday afternoon, over nineteen hours since I had left. I had covered the best part of 110km, with about 6000m of positive altitude change, and I looked like I had brought most of the trail with me. I was caked in mud, still with as many layers of clothing on as during the night, the day had been shrouded in fog so any morale boosting sunlight together with the impressive views of the mountains, remained a pipe dream. I had taken off one of my beanies.

My right ankle was more than 50% bigger than it was when I had left the start line, and my socks were more hole than sock as they had taken such a pounding whilst having spent nineteen hours soaking wet. I had planned on a change of clothes, particularly socks, but given the last minute nature of the route change the drop bags with my spare gear remained in Courmayeur, a town I had yet to visit.

I ran into Chamonix with a couple of people hot on my heels, and from nowhere I managed to sprint the last couple of kilometres through the village. People were cheering me, runners that had already completed the race, families, nutters, whoever they were it didn't matter, it all served to give me that all important adrenaline rush. It had not come a moment too soon, but I turned the last corner of the race to the finish line, and as I crossed I felt an overwhelming sense of relief.

I picked up my blue finisher's gilet, recognised and coveted the world over, and immediately felt a sense of loss. This was more than the usual post race depression – the feeling of having had a certain goal in mind for so long and focussing on that one specific goal to the detriment of other aspects of one's life that when the goal has been realised it leaves a hole, a sense of loss and mourning. I was experiencing something more. The tenth edition of the UTMB would always be known as a short and different route. Certain aspects of it made it challenging, but it wasn't the actual UTMB. As I hobbled back to my guest house to try and get the grime off me before heading home, I felt I still had unfinished business.

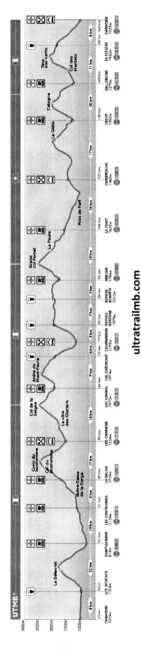

ultratrailmb.com

151

Saturday 20 June 2014, Cro Magnon

As I reached the town of Tende, Sonia, Paola and Luca were there to greet me, and seemed a little surprised when I just grabbed a little water for my back pack and headed straight out the checkpoint. I was one of the last to reach the checkpoint and was all too aware of the time limits, having beaten this one by a matter of minutes. I had been taking things very steady to conserve energy as I knew that the journey to the start had taken an enormous amount of my reserves from me. I had also struggled on the downhill, technical section, into Tende. Each time my foot hit the ground, a tiny chafing of the sock on already tender feet was adding to the agony. A shudder of pain would also go through each quad, just above the knee, as my overworked shock absorbers were struggling with the renewed punishment.

My main concern was beating the cut offs and whilst I could afford to be slow I could not afford to waste any time at checkpoints sitting down and resting. As I left a faintly bewildered crew behind I trotted up a tree lined avenue, the sun pooling on the floor. It looked like it was going to be a hot one, which had positives and negatives. The heat might cause my feet to swell, compounding any damage, and also slowing progress generally. However, it promised to open up some spectacular vistas, a large part of what I actually enjoyed about ultra running. Not to mention the distraction from internal travails I might be wrestling with.

I was not disappointed. A few kilometres later I headed up a steep mountain path, and as I looked over the valley I was afforded a view of a mill, a kilometre or so in the distance. There was a beautiful flower garden surrounding a pond so flat it was like a mirror, reflecting the reds, yellows and mauves of the flowers. The mill house itself must have been five hundred years old, shade afforded by some ancient tree. A man was working in the garden, perhaps digging vegetables or weeding, too far away to tell. It was like something that Monet or Constable would have painted, and I was amazed it was actually in the French – Italian mountains, rather than in the Cotswolds or Normandie; it looked so out of place.

Once back above the tree line, I was in much more familiar territory. The footpath was so narrow it was one person wide, and appeared to have been cut into the rock by a pizza slicer. I stuck close to the side of the mountain as one wrong foot could see me plunging thousands of metres down. Every time I rounded a bend I could see several kilometres into the distance, the path plainly visible in the scrub and rock. The path roughly followed a ridge in the mountain range, and the views to my right were amazing and vast once I had gotten over the dizzying height. Verdant valleys, jagged, grey mountain spikes, the odd wisp of mist carpeting a valley floor.

To my left was a different picture. A few metres above the path, the top of the ridge heralded a thick, rolling duvet of fog, threatening to spill over onto the precarious path. To navigate the path in clear sunshine was tricky enough, notwithstanding fatigue, loose rocks and boulders threatening to trip and tip me over the edge. To then reduce the visibility to virtually nothing would have probably stopped my Cro Magnon attempt in its tracks, given my precarious hold on the time barriers.

The other added excitement of this path was that it encountered part of the Maginot line. After World War One, and the visible expansionary and military policies of several fascist governments in the 1920's and 30's, France decided to build a virtual wall of defense from North to South to keep everyone out. The border with Italy, with the fascist government in power, was obviously seen as needing some bolstering. Instead of actually building a wall, they built the Maginot line, named for its inventor, where there would be strategic defences each covering an arc, such that the arcs overlapped. In this way the line was supposed to be impregnable. Of course, the reality was that the Germans just came round the North and the Italians in the South, and as a result the Maginot line itself remains broadly intact. The path I was on intersected with some of the defences, in reality a network of tunnels and caves cut into the rock itself. Occasionally the path would give way to a rotting grate – perhaps an access hatch or an air duct; treacherous if one slipped into it and trapped a foot, and potentially even worse. The Maginot line looked inherently more dangerous to a unsuspecting trail runner than it had proved hazardous to the Fascists in the 1930's. Some of the holes were wide enough for a person, and so deep I could not make out the bottom. It would have been easy to plunge into them, never to be seen again.

The organisers had done their best to mark out the hazards with reflective tape, but add in a little fog and I would have doubtlessly buckled, even if I had made it to the cut offs.

I jogged on, traversing the ridge just before the fog enveloped us all. The trail had descended to the tree line, and I was in a thickly wooded area. I had been joined by a fellow runner, and we swapped stories for a bit before the next aid station. He was a nurse, and was intrigued by the diabetes narrative to my story. We chatted for a bit about that, in broken French and English and whatever Italian I had picked up the night before (it seemed like an age). He had tried the Cro Magnon the previous year but had given up. He said his body had been fine but he had lost the mental strength. He was hopeful this year would be his year. He certainly seemed strong as we ran between two rows of bombed out barracks, remnants of a World War. It didn't strike me until later the poignancy that British, French, Italians and quite probably Germans were all undertaking the same endeavour side by side in a place which had seen our forbears pitted against each other in two bloody wars.

I was struggling physically to keep up with the nurse, so I tapped him on the back and ushered him on. I could not afford to go out too hard and then have nothing later on, so I did the prudent thing, although I think he liked the company.

Only a couple of kilometres further on I reached a mountain refuge which had been taken over by the organisers as an aid station. The moisture in the air made it very cold, and I grabbed some Coke and water and walked through. I saw my temporary trail buddy sitting down, sipping at some hot soup. He raised his Styrofoam cup to me in salute and I could see in his eyes that he was beaten. Not even a third of the race done, feeling guilty, I tried to chivvy him along, urging him to join me. I wasn't aiming for a speed record, just to complete. But he refused all overtures, and I had my own cut offs to think of.

I used the downhill after the aid station to gently jog, readjusting my back pack as I did so. A medical badged Land Rover was parked just off the cinder trails, and I heard a lot of yelling. Four runners were surrounding the ambulance and getting in. They looked physically fine, but the brutality of the course had already mentally taken its toll and they were calling it a day. I wished there was a way I could have transplanted their legs and feet instead of mine, but I won't deny that seeing them cave long before me was a morale booster in itself.

29 June 2013, Western States 100 Best laid plans....

I buckled over with the pain of a second massive contraction starting in my lower stomach and moving in slow motion upwards, until it gurgled into my throat expelling nothing but air and bile out of my mouth. The trajectory the nausea had taken was in parallel to my own journey from the bottom of the stiflingly hot canyon between Last Chance and Devil's Thumb.

Temperatures had registered 102 F / 38.8 C at Auburn, the second highest official temperature recorded for the race in 40 years. The combination of no wind, little shade, and a creek at the bottom of the canyon adding to the trapped humidity, I was all too aware that the heat in the canyon was significantly higher. Coupled with an ascent (which, although not technical, was devilishly steep) after 47 miles of running, it was no wonder my body was protesting. I had lost a lot of weight in the first 30 miles of the race, indicating dehydration, and was aware of back pain which could have just been back pain, but could also have been a sign of kidney distress and possible renal failure on the horizon. This was not the time to start vomiting and ensure more dehydration and perhaps throw away my whole race. It was definitely time to put any lingering thoughts I had of a silver buckle to one side, and just get on with finishing. I pulled myself together as far as I could, and covered the last 200 metres to the Devil's Thumb aid station for another weigh in, and some well earned ministrations from the extremely kind hearted volunteers so characteristic along the whole course.

This was the second hottest Western States 100 ever, with the California heatwave recording the hottest ever temperatures seen in the USA. At the race briefing, the organisers had told us to put aside thoughts of times and splits, and just to run a safe race. I just had the strategy to start slow and not only hope that my body would hold for the full 100.2 miles. After all, a few months before I had been hanging from my seat belt, upside down facing the wrong way on a dual carriageway.

19 January 2013, The Whole World Turned Upside Down

"She's hit us!" I exclaimed involuntarily, as I felt a huge bang on the right rear wing of my truck. I steered into the skid, turning the wheel hard to the left, full lock, as the back end was wrested away from me. All I could hear was the scraping of the windscreen wipers on the glass moving in slow motion, until a sound like an explosion as the back left of the car hit the barrier separating the two carriageways. A gut wrenching tearing noise followed for a few seconds, as the fender scraped along the wall whilst the steering wheel writhed and twisted in my hands like an angry snake.

"Daddy, what have you done?" I heard my terrified ten year old daughter, Alice, scream from the back seat, as we careered headfirst into a wall on the inside of the dual carriageway at fifty kilometres per hour. Fleeting thoughts that any damage could be polished out were replaced by "Oh my God we're all going to die".

I felt a huge fist hit me in the face and a nano-second later realised it was the airbag as it crumpled, having done its job. Events were happening so fast my brain couldn't keep up. Glass flew at me from all directions, and I felt the tugging at my shoulder before I could register it was scraping up the road. The truck had been tossed over by the multiple impacts and momentum, and was now no more than a Matchbox toy.

"IS EVERYONE OK?" I shouted, as I turned off the ignition to stop the deafening noise of the car alarm going off, and tried not to panic as the cabin filled with smoke. The car had come to rest facing the wrong way on the dual carriageway. On the driver's side door handles. I could hear screaming from the back, but I was dreading what I was going to find. Alice was directly behind me and if my shoulder had been dragged up the road what state was her head going to be in? I had gone from having a lovely chat with my kids and looking forward to a roast chicken Saturday lunch, to being in the middle of a very loud and painful nightmare in the space of a heartbeat.

I undid my seat belt, fell onto my left side, and frantically turned around and saw two very very frightened little faces on my back seat, tears making tracks through the blood on their cheeks. My eldest, Emily, had already managed to undo her seat belt, and as she was behind the passenger seat she had been suspended in the air as if from a roller coaster that had stopped half way through a loop.

"EMILY! GET OFF ME!"

"I'm trying Alice. Look, just let me put my hand..."

"OW! That's my ARM!"

Emily had fallen onto Alice once she had managed to unclip the seat belt, and despite everything normal service had resumed: bickering siblings. I knew they couldn't be too badly hurt. Thank God.

As quickly as I could (mindful of the smoke floating around the car) I found firm footing amongst all the broken glass and debris on the floor, and I tried to open the door. It was harder than I had been expecting; I was not tall enough to really get it open, and it weighed a ton. I could only open it a crack, and the kids were going to need my help to get out. All of a sudden, it was wrested from me, further shocking me in my confused state. A passer-by had stopped and was holding it open; I hurled the kids one after the other out the car, and they were helped to the roadside. I was weightless as I pulled myself out after them and hustled them away to safety, before dealing with the aftermath of the crash.

Aside from some minor cuts and more major bruises, we were all relatively unscathed. The adrenaline was providing anaesthetic for the worst of the visible cuts and bruises, and that which we could not see.

My wife arrived with our third and youngest daughter, and took all three off to a kindly householder nearby to escape the freezing rain. Once the kids had gone, my legs lost the ability to support me; my composure disappeared. The rain mingled with my tears. I thanked God for the hundredth time that the kids were ok. The ambulance crew suggested we should be x-rayed if any pain persisted, but on the face of it we all seemed to be ok.

We calmed down after a nice meal, hot bath and liberal applications of antiseptic and arnica, and eventually went to bed, but between my own shock and the kids' flashbacks, sleep was elusive. After a morning spent filling out forms and dealing with the more bureaucratic side of the accident, we went off to hospital for some x-rays, as we all had a great deal of neck, shoulder, and arm pain. I struggled to hold a pen to sign the insurance forms, the pain was so bad.

The kids were at the forefront of my mind, but once it became apparent that there was only bruising and whiplash, my next thought was the Western States 100 miler in June, and whether I would be able to train for it.

The Western States 100 Mile Endurance Run is "the world's oldest and most prestigious 100 mile trail race", according to their website. The race starts in Squaw Valley, Lake Tahoe, and ends in Auburn, California. The idea is to traverse the mountain paths in under thirty hours. The race has been run since 1974 when Gordy Ainsleigh entered the Tevis Cup horse race, on foot, and completed the course in under 24 hours. Over time, the horse and foot races parted company, and the Western States 100 Mile Endurance Run grew in stature and popularity year by year. The course has 18000 feet (5500 metres) of elevation gain, and 23000 feet (7000 metres) of descent, making the course one of the toughest in the world due to altitude and temperature changes. The field is limited to around 400 runners, due to National Parks legislation, and as a result entry has been oversubscribed since 1979. The entry process is very strict – for my part, I had to qualify through my finishing time at the Ultra Trail of Mont Blanc in 2012, no mean feat in itself, and then go through a lottery process as each qualifying place has more than fifteen applicants. I entered with the very realistic expectation of not getting a place, but the running gods smiled on me and I was very lucky to receive an entry in the ballot. To say I was shocked is an understatement.

Not only was the entry ticket rarer than hen's teeth [if you weren't brought up in the country then you might not know, but hens generally don't have teeth], but then I had to negotiate taking a week off from family responsibilities as the race coincided with the end of term and all the associated shows and parents evenings and all that fun stuff parents know and love. When I mentioned how hard it was to get a place, how lucky I was to get an entry, and how I would organise baby sitting with both sets of grandparents, my kids urged me to go, and my wife very kindly volunteered to crew for me. I booked flights and a nice hotel so that we could have a nice break together, even if I was going to eschew one of those nights in luxury to spend it on the mountain trails.

After all that, the last thing I needed was for several "what ifs" to come together in succession and stop me going to the Western States. A momentary loss of traction at exactly the wrong moment from another driver and my journey to California was in jeopardy. I prayed it hadn't ruined my chances of participating in one of the most prestigious and exclusive ultra marathons in the entire world.

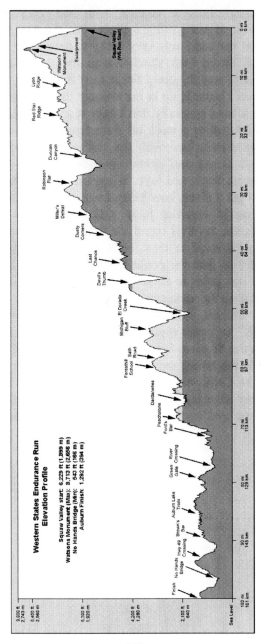

Western States Endurance Run
Elevation Profile

Squaw Valley start: 6,229 ft (1,899 m)
Watsons Monument (Max): 8,713 ft (2,656 m)
No Hands Bridge (Min): 543 ft (166 m)
Auburn Finish: 1,292 ft (394 m)

WSER.org

162

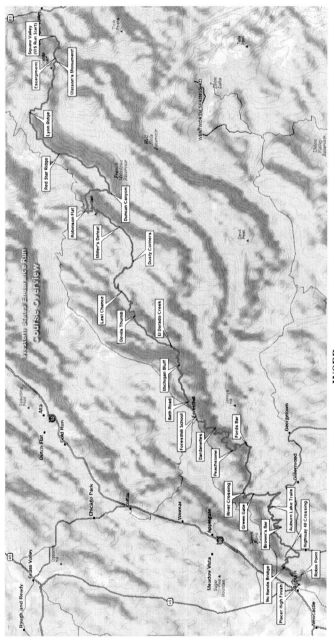

WSER.org

29 June 2013, Western States 100

After the car crash I had battled various little niggles, both mental and physical. The stiff neck had dissipated after a couple of weeks but an occasional calf strain or lower back pain would crop up, which was completely out of the ordinary for me. It had also taken me several months to get over the mental trauma of the accident. The inevitable "what ifs" that played out in my dreams, and I would awake with the image of one or both of the kids covered in blood and unresponsive; images that just wouldn't go away. I became much quicker to anger and was involved in shouting matches with people in traffic, or even on the street, over trivial issues.

I wasn't sure that over the extended and rough race that a muscular weakness caused by the crash or hiccup in training might end up with a race ending injury. Or I was having doubts that I was mentally strong enough to get through the race. My strategy was to start at a comfortable pace well within my limitations, to maximise the chances of finishing, and hopefully leave something in the tank for the latter stages.

The race started at altitude, which in itself would increase energy usage, as my heart rate would be unusually elevated in the early stages of the race. Due to parental responsibilities, Mrs R and I were not able to travel to California until three days before the race, where two weeks would have been optimal to adjust to the time zone and altitude.

However, I did what I could to acclimate, going on the trek to Emigrant Pass. This would be the top of the first climb of the race: 2550 feet / 850m of altitude gain in around four miles / six kilometres, taking us to around 8500 feet / 2850 metres above sea level. An introduction to the history of the race was held at High Noon at the Watson Memorial which marked the top of Emigrant pass and the start of the race proper.

I hoped that light exercise would accelerate acclimation, and coupled that with a lovely ride on single speed fat tyre rental bikes in a stunning shade of pink, following the local river from our hotel, and enjoying an icy dip along the way.

The whole atmosphere of Squaw Valley was fizzing with excitement during the lead up to the race, with plenty of other runners in evidence by their sinewy limbs and faded finisher's t-shirts from other races such as Mount Fuji or Leadville.

Part of the attraction of the Western States Endurance Race was because of its enduring and interesting history. It was the first 100 mile foot race, and the way it started was by accident. There had been a horse race called the Tevis Cup running since 1955, which started to keep alive the Western States Trail used by goldminers for several hundred years and probably Native Americans for eons before that. In 1974, Gordy Ainsleigh, a 27 year old Tevis Veteran, had entered the horse race but shortly before the race, his mount went lame. He sought permission, which was subsequently granted, to enter the race on foot. To everyone's disbelief, he finished within the allotted time (24 hours), and the foot race was born. The following year Gordy entered on foot again, this time with a friend, Ron Kelley, who became the first DNF (Did Not Finish). The following year crewed his buddy Cowman Amooha, who finished but in 24 hours and 30 minutes, just past the cut off. Over the years that followed the entries snowballed until the original Tevis Cup horse race and the new Western States 100 went their separate ways. The foot race became so popular that the impact on the National Park needed to be taken into consideration, and annual entries were capped by the authorities at 400, including Gordy Ainsleigh who was always Number 0, in perpetuity.

It was pretty exciting and emotional at the start, and everyone was swept up in it, including Mrs R who was usually only seen up at 3am if she hadn't been to bed! I chatted to a few guys I had met including Gary from

Montreal (although originally GB), and Dan from close to Auburn (near the finish) and then we were off, walking up the first climb from around 1900m to around 2700m in 6km. If anyone says the Western States is all downhill, they are lying!

I spent most of the first climb chatting to other runners, my accent pointing me out as an international entrant and giving us something to talk about. Each runner's number also had their nationality represented by the three letter acronym such as USA or GBR. Mine had MCO which again was a bit of a talking point. Apparently I was the first runner ever from Monaco, and a feature of my race was the reaction of the volunteers at the aid stations trying to work out what MCO stood for, and me trying to explain it whilst battling ever increasing fatigue, and other issues.

I managed to meet Gordy and we exchanged a few words before I pulled away from him. 67 years old, and 27 finishes! I also saw Cowman, wearing his trademark horned hat, a throwback from his personal celebration of the America's bicentennial in 1976 when he ran through the streets of Lake Tahoe wearing nothing but the horned helmet and body paint.

As I crested the peak and gave a nod to the now familiar Watson's Monument, I looked back and was rewarded with a spectacular sunrise. Wisps of mist were rising off the water in the valley, with the first twinkles of pink and orange sun visible on the surface of Lake Tahoe. I headed off into the first 30 miles and first serious canyon, with my crew, Mrs R, meeting me at the top of it. It was still chilly, and we headed through mountain pastures full of unseasonal wild flowers due to the recent rain, and then some overgrown scrubby brush where we traced a muddy creek bed in single file.

The sun was gently warming us and with only patchy cover due to the previous year's forest fires, it wasn't long before the sun became a serious issue. I tried to drink regularly from my water bladder, and took water melon at the frequent aid stations, enjoying the carnival atmosphere of the race and admiring the landmarks I had only read about.

I just followed the beautiful trail in an easy relaxed manner, letting others pull ahead if they wanted. I tried to keep my fluids up with the augmented water in my pouch, but it was quite hard to judge it. I had been using the same electrolyte and carb infused powder for years, and I had brought spare powders with me.

I passed a couple of runners sitting down at the first marathon mark, 26 miles / 42 kilometres, and had to focus on the goal to avoid joining them. I found that I was drinking more than I had expected and was swiftly going through my powders, but as I pulled in to the 30 mile aid station at Robinson Flat I was feeling shattered after a long hot climb out of Duncan Canyon.

We had been weighed at the check in, and I had been around 169 pounds / 76 kilos, then again at the start - 170.2 pounds / 77 kilos. The organisers liked to monitor runners for signs of over or de-hydration, and I was due for the first in-race weigh in at Robinson Flat. The aid station itself was a sort of camp site and picnic area, full to bursting with white camper vans or "RV's" in local parlance. The trail itself was roped off, with spectators cheering every runner as we jogged into view. I glimpsed Mrs R trying to squeeze her way to the front, and she tried to chat, but I was having a dark moment, not sure whether I was going to complete the race at all, as I felt weak, puffed, and hot.

I shocked the aid station staff, and myself, when they found out I had gone down to 162 pounds / 73.5 kilos. I tried to push on through and continue to run after my water supply was replenished, but was told to sit, and when I protested, I was shoved into a deck chair. The aid station staff watched over me whilst I drank several beakers of Coke and water, and after a few slices of watermelon and apple, my spirits slowly started to lift.

After I had regained enough weight to satisfy the aid station volunteers, Mrs R grabbed me and took me under her wing applying vaseline, sun lotion, and making sure I had all the fluids I needed. Within a few minutes I was off into a gloriously wooded and shaded mile and my mood and physical state were lifted by a factor of several thousand percent.

Which was just as well because the next section was fire affected forest and hill side facing directly into the blazing sun. Great swathes of forest had been wiped out by the fires, and the only vegetation was the odd sapling or shrub. Vicious looking toothpicks punctuating the skyline. The sun was high overhead, and it was hot. Very hot.

I continued along the trail, jogging when I could and walking when my body told me it had to, and was caught up by three red t-shirted security patrollers. These runners were part of the organisation that ran sections of the trail administering to runners in difficulty, and providing moral support to others. These were two men, both firefighters, who had met last year at the race. One of them had run the race, and the other had been a pacer and crew for someone else, but as his runner had dropped out part way through, he had stepped in as a pacer for the other one at the last minute. It was clear they were now firm friends.

Elke was the third, a local born and bred, and she too had run the race the previous year. She was part of the Western States Trail management team and the trail was in her blood. It was great to have some company on this challenging, undulating, but predominantly downhill section, with someone prodding me to drink regularly.

I had been a little shaken up by the weight loss, and I also had some pain in my lower back. Having experienced renal pain in the past, I still wasn't sure whether the back pain was muscular or internal. Perhaps fatigue and stiffness were setting in, or in fact dehydration was affecting my kidneys. I kept a close eye on the colour of my urine, and regularly did the pinch test on the back of my hand. As my urine gradually lightened, the pain dissipated.

I certainly needed all my energies and concentration, because we were approaching the first of the notorious series of canyons, infamous because they were so sheltered and humid. The registered temperature had been 102 F / 39 C in the open, but the canyons were like huge outdoor saunas with little shelter, no breeze, and the added bonus of a light creek at the bottom allowing the water to evaporate, which increased the humidity. Whatever the temperature outside, you could guarantee it would be a good 10-20 degrees more in the canyons. Couple that with quad busting descents, morale sapping ascents, and they were often the graveyard of many a Western States entrant's dreams and goals.

I breezed through Last Chance, a mining ghost town. I tried to remember my avid research before the race but the origins of the name were murky. Supposedly two early prospectors were days away from the nearest town, out of supplies, and down to their last rifle bullet. They stalked a deer, and as the better shot took aim, the other said something like "You'd better not miss. This is our last chance." Whether true or not, it made for a great distraction from the overall discomfort of being 43 miles into a trail race, and still having 57 more to go.

To that point I was just ticking off the miles, and my descent into the first of the canyons went pretty well, even though the descent was at times technical with steep switchbacks and loose rocks. I had read about people trashing their quads in the first half of the race and subsequently DNF'ing, but all my quad training from Mad Dog Mike paid off as I passed a few people.

But the climb up was a different story. I used the river at the bottom, and picturesque waterfall which I took full advantage of to soak myself. It was just as well, the ascent was like the retreat from Stalingrad! It was very steep, and people were buckling right from the beginning, littering the track with broken bodies. I ended up leading a veritable *peloton* up the hill to Devils Thumb, providing encouraging words and motivation to myself as much to the others.

Then it all became too much for me, and a huge convulsion gripped me from the inside; I bent double, and dry heaved bringing up nothing but bile. Unfortunately I was right next to the medics, sent in advance by the aid station, and I tried to retch as nonchalantly as I could for fear of having my number plucked off me and being disqualified. The medics, however, didn't seem overly bothered (having seen far worse), and I dragged myself to the aid station and passed the weigh in and cognitive test with, surprisingly, flying colours!

I had a chance to look around whilst my water bladder was filled with water, my powders and ice, and whilst I had suffered there were indeed more people in much worse shape than me. Several people were asleep or unconscious on military looking cots, and another couple sitting looking distinctly zombie like, being ministered to by medics. I can see why they didn't bat an eyelid when I had a couple of pathetic dry heaves. I felt positively athletic in comparison. One poor chap, Dan, had actually passed out on the trail and fallen down the hill, but had managed to pull himself together and get up the hill to recover over time in the aid station.

I had clearly put too much into the climb, so took my time at the aid station to rehydrate and have some more watermelon. I had never been offered this in a race before, but it was like manna, sweet and wet. I gobbled down a few chunks, and shuffled on my way, kicking up dust as I went.

"Hey how are you doing?"

"Not great, actually."

"Sorry to hear that. I'm Ben. What's the problem?"

Compared to the canyon I was in much better shape, the trees giving natural shade, ice in my hat and cooling my quads trapped by the lycra shorts I was wearing. My spirits had been lifted by the comparison to the other guys "resting" at the aid station. However, it was still a little unfamiliar for me to be offering advice to a fellow runner, amateur as I considered myself to be.

"Oh hi, I'm Esther. My thighs really hurt, just here." She pointed to her quads. I had read about the Western States and the toll it took on people's legs as the descent was a lot greater overall than the ascent. I had trained accordingly with Mad Dog, but had quite a bit of previous experience in shorter races with descents. Ever since Psycho made me look like a numpty way back in 2007 in Gorbio.

Esther was pointing to her quads, and I suggested she did as I did. I slowed to chat to her whilst she discretely transferred some ice from her bottles down her shorts, and it was a nice diversion which took my mind off the fact I was only just over half way. Eventually I pulled ahead of Esther and wished her well. I never saw her pass me again, although I noticed on the web results she finished, and strongly.

"Hey mate, loving the matching outfit!" I yelled out as the Jolly Green Giant overtook me at speed. I was jogging, using the gentle downhill to get a bit of speed up, but he was thundering down the slope looking very strong. He slowed just enough to tell me that he had bought all his gear the day before as he was from cooler climes and was not used to the excessive heat. The only colour they had in his enormous size was bright green. And then he was off kicking up clouds of dust with every footfall.

At the next aid station, I stopped briefly to empty my shoes of trail, and of course bumped into the ever present Elke to say hi. I was pleased to get past the landmark rock, the Devil's Thumb and I whooped as we passed the half way mark just after the historic Deadwood Cemetery entrance. With visions of toy holsters and plastic spurs as a kid, I managed to resist the temptation to pop in for a nose around!

At the bottom of the canyon, I immersed myself as much as possible in the creek, to about half way up my shins which left a tide mark of dirt on my legs. The water level was exceptionally low, even for the time of year, but even so the cooling water felt fabulous on my body and soul, and I dunked my cap before heading out of the canyon.

Climbs, descents, dusty trails, aid stations with ice down the shorts and in the cap all blended into one. Every footstep was a step closer to the finish, and it was as much about enjoying the experience, runners and volunteers alike, as it was a race.

I took a moment to savour finishing with the Canyons as I crested the top of the hill. I knew Mrs R would be meeting me at the Michigan Bluff aid station at 55 miles. The dirt gave way to tarmac, indicating approaching civilisation, and I travelled about half a mile / 800 metres on a road as a whisper became a faint cheer and then a constant roar, rising and falling. I rounded a corner and at least 50 people were standing and cheering behind a plastic tape.

The funny thing was that I couldn't see who they would be cheering for. I looked around to check if anyone was behind me, perhaps an elite athlete or a celebrity but there was no one; the road was clear in front of me too. It dawned on me that they may actually be cheering for me. I pointed at myself and then raised both palms skywards, and they cheered harder. I was overcome with emotion at these people whom I had never met, nor would likely again, just standing there enjoying the race. Whether they held ambitions to do it, or just admired anyone that tried it, they were caught up in it too. I managed a little bow to the crowd's amusement and more cheers and clapping.

I trotted into Michigan Bluff, a tiny little hamlet with its ranks of houses swelled by the phalanx of RV's lining both sides of the road. I was guided into a tent for the obligatory weigh in and passed with flying colours. Whilst I was stood on the scales someone grabbed my pack and filled it with water. I was met by Mrs R, fully into her role of crew, as she grabbed my arm and led me to her "station". She had settled between two massive RV's, both with small tubs filled with ice outside them, several people milling around with various food, gels, clothes and drinks, waiting for their runners.

Mrs R had laid everything that she could think that I might need out for me on a towel, electrolyte powders, protein bars, trail mix, spare socks, Coke and water. She sat me down on a rock, took my shoes off and emptied out the stones. Uncomfortable with being served like royalty, I tried to reach down to my feet to untie my own laces, but I felt an early twinge of cramp in both calves. I sat back and let Mrs R do the honours. My shoes continually picked up bits of trail, dirt, stones and twigs which were causing havoc with the soles of my feet, and we figured it better to remove the offending items before they became a more serious problem.

Shoes emptied and morale lifted, I set off; it was getting cooler, and whilst I had no idea of the time it was still very much daylight. I had planned on picking up a headlamp at 62 miles at the Foresthill Aid station which I had calculated, whilst sitting at my desk back in Europe, that I should reach with a nice buffer of daylight before it got dark. Mrs R had a spare just in case, and also for her personal use whilst schlepping from various laybys and car parks to the aid stations. The plan seemed to be working pretty well despite the brief bout of nausea and general aches and pains, so I decided to stick to our/my plan and pick up the headlamps at Foresthill, seven miles / nine kilometres hence.

Michigan Bluff was the first aid station where runners could pick up pacers, so not only was I passing or being passed by runners, it became little groups of two or more rather than individuals. I was in a minority of one, as the vast majority of runners had utilised the pacer rule, and I could see why. During the hours of dusk and early night, the body tends to shut down, the body clock expecting a person to slow down after the work day and relax before going to sleep. I knew from experience that these hours were dangerous; the runner might lose the mental ability to carry on and quit; or perhaps a momentary lapse of concentration could result in a fall or trip and the race would be over due to injury. I completely understood why people had pacers, but I had never used one and as it was just the two of us travelling to the far side of the US from Europe, I had a very small pool of people from which to choose.

I was making good time down the descent to Bath Road, on single track through the woods. I felt good and the cooler air was helping me move a little more fluidly, and faster. A sub twenty four finish was almost beyond reach, but a tiny part of me thought that if I hustled at a fast clip all the way to the finish and the terrain was forgiving enough, it might still be possible.

And then someone switched out the lights. There was no warning. One minute it was light, the next dark.

We were still in the mountains even though the path was not as technical as the Alps, and, true to form in the mountains, the light disappeared with no warning. I blinked, my eyes trying to adjust and utilising what little light I could glean from the moon, and I continued on slowly. As my eyes became more and more used to the light, and the moon gradually showed its face, I was actually able to jog a bit, hoping that I wouldn't trip over a root or bump into something I really didn't want to bump into (bears, snakes, mountain lions, and poisonous stinging plants were tops of the list). I was still about a mile or two from Bath Road, and despite the lack of illumination, managed to make up a couple more places. One chap I passed was broken despite having two pacers chivvying him along with encouraging and firm words. They all had headlamps which would have lit up a football game lighting the trail ahead, and were chatting so loudly they neither saw nor heard me approaching from the rear. As I brushed past them all three jumped into the air, the runner perhaps slightly less spritely.

"Hey man, where's your torch?" the runner asked as I jogged ahead, his pacers wisely suggesting he focus on his own race and not mine.

"Foresthill," I replied.

"Here take mine, I have a spare."

"Dave, come on, you might need it, keep it." His pacer shushed him.

But he insisted.

"No it's ok, I have this one, you have one each, we have batteries, he has none. It's trail karma dude."

"Just leave it at the next aid station," he said as he handed me a headlamp.

"Thanks mate. I really appreciate it."

I made a mental note of his number so that I could tell the volunteers when I got to Bath Road, but was still pondering how to continue onwards to Foresthill with no torch. I knew that I could use the "Force" for only so long before my luck ran out and at the very least took a wrong turn, not something I relished.

"Oh hi Ben, how are you doing?" I turned from the volunteer I was giving the headlamp to, and was confronted with Elke, contentedly munching on a pizza and chatting to a friend, at the trestle table that marked the Bath Road aid station.

"Um, great thanks Elke. I...erm...well..." I stuttered, feeling like a complete pillock.

"You won't believe me if I told you." I shook my head, embarrassed.

"But I managed to pack a headlamp in my drop bag at Foresthill, and Mrs R has my other one."

Without a word, she managed to stuff the rest of the pizza in her mouth in a completely lady-like fashion, grabbed her sidekick, and they set off either side of me, like Police outriders. They accompanied me, illuminating my way in stereo all the way to Foresthill at 62 miles.

Elke had previously mentioned that her daughter Chloe was excited about being a pacer for one of their friends who had managed to secure a coveted spot, but she thought that the runner was struggling early on in the race. Having completed the race herself previously, she espoused the merits of having a pacer, and a local one at that, for encouragement, support, directions and rudimentary medical advice if needed. There was a chance that Chloe would be looking for another runner if hers had dropped, as she was particularly looking forward to the river crossing at mile 78 / 120 kilometres.

As soon as we arrived at Foresthill, Mrs R, slightly puzzled at my escort although relieved I had made it to the aid station without a torch, greeted me, loaded me up with two headlamps, spare batteries, bars, electrolytes and all the bits that she knew I would need. In the meantime, Elke borrowed a walkie talkie and quickly established that Chloe's runner had DNF'd due to injury. Having had it impressed on me, I recognised the wisdom of having a pacer, particularly a combat medic with local knowledge, and Chloe and I were introduced. If the roles had been reversed I am not sure I would have accepted with as much gusto as Chloe, given the liberal coating of dirt and sweat and other unknown substances, as well as my hollow eyes and slightly garbled speech pattern.

The race organisers were geared up to pacers, having invented the concept all the way back when Gordy and Cowman had pioneered the race in the 1970's. They had a spare pacers bib for every runner at Foresthill as lots of runners, and sometimes even their pacers, would have dropped out. Chloe changed her pacer's bib to match mine, and was thrilled to be given the opportunity to run. I sensed she was particularly excited about the river crossing at mile 78, the famous and photogenic Rucky Chucky crossing.

Chloe was well prepared, something you would expect from a combat medic in the National Guard with a tour of Iraq under her belt. She had stocked up on salt tabs, batteries, M&M's, and other stuff, for her planned runner, but of course I was on my own plan so just had bits of apple, protein bar, melon and my powders. We made up some really good time because we both seemed to like downhills, the heat had subsided, and her local knowledge was second to none warning me in great detail about upcoming terrain such as deep sand, technical sections, or even just boosting my morale by knowing how long a climb would be.

It may have been the night, the fatigue, or just the topography but we seemed to turn left a lot, every switchback, junction, corner was a left turn. It became a running joke that we would just end up back at Foresthill! Every aid station was breezed through; Chloe even emptied my shoes of rocks for me (not a job I'd like at the best of times let alone in the middle of the night and after I'd covered some 70 miles of dirt trail and multiple creek crossings), and we overtook heaps of people as we moved through the checkpoints smoothly whilst others would be sitting, lying or even sleeping. We ran all the downs, some of the flats and walked the ups, but I was very pleased I was still able to move forward after the tough day.

At 78 miles, we reached the river crossing, a highlight of the run. Whilst there had been a lot of creeks and streams, this was neck deep and the organisers had laid a rope across it with helpers in wet suits to guide runners across. For Chloe this was the bit she had been looking forward to; she had been waxing lyrically about the steps hewn into the cliff face and how beautiful it was. I agreed that they looked beautiful, but my legs were not happy with the physical demands of descending an actual staircase, no matter how stunning it looked.

Per usual, it was well organised with aid stations on either side of the river, music playing, fairy lights, and Chloe began telling everybody that I was the first runner from Monaco, which created some excitement. The river crossing itself was magical, but also bloody chilly - good for the muscles!

On the other side, Elke and Chloe's boyfriend Sal met us and we hiked to the top of the brief climb, saying our goodbyes. Elke had finished her security patrol, been home for a shower, changed and come out to meet us. She didn't know me from Adam and was there to provide support, knowledge, and friendship not just to pick up her daughter who was pacing me! I was so grateful for all their help, I didn't think I would have made it as far as I had without it.

We reached the next checkpoint, the third in quick succession, and with a little trepidation about my prospects on both sides, I turned right back onto the trail.

"Dude, just follow the trail, and after about a mile turn left. DO NOT MISS THE LEFT TURN."

A young, confident chap from the aid station with a garland of flowers around his neck, straw hat, and loud Hawaiian t-shirt and shorts jogged with me for a couple of hundred metres, explaining the trail and important junctions. Because of him I was able to continue in confidence and did not miss the important left turn. The constant barrage of kindness and selflessness from these complete strangers was almost overwhelming, and I was pleased to have a moment to myself to gather myself together. Mentally, as well as physically, the race was taking its toll.

I was running on my own again, in the mountains, at night, and it was magical. Whole hours would go by when I wouldn't see any other runners, until one passed, or I passed them, all with herds of pacers. I was running well until a huge balloon welled up in my stomach. I stopped, pulled to one side of the track and thought I was going to vomit. The balloon gradually made its way up from my stomach, up and up to my throat and then out my mouth. A huge burp came out. But the balloon in my stomach remained. I felt bloated, but couldn't vomit or burp again. Then the hiccups began. Great big racking hiccups. And then little chirping noises like baby birds waiting to be fed. I thought it might have been the constant sugary water and electrolytes, Coke, trail mix and protein bars. But I had had all that before. There must have been something I hadn't tried before.

That was it. Watermelon. It tasted so good going down, sweet and moist. But my body was not used to it, and couldn't process it on the move. It was all just sitting there like a malign passenger, in my stomach. The constant hiccups were a reminder to never try anything new during a race again.

20 June 2014, Cro Magnon No Easy Path

I had nothing left. I staggered a few more steps on the cinder trail, located a large rock, and sat down, exhausted. That was it. My race was over. I couldn't go any further. I hadn't even gotten to Breil Sur Roya, marking the approximate half way point, but I was busted both mentally and physically. I felt like a deflated tyre, in every way.

I wearily unclipped my pack and tried to get comfortable on my rock, my lycra shorts providing me little protection from the cold, unforgiving stone. I was in a wood, the path wide enough for a tractor to get down, permanent evidence of the multiple wars littering both sides of the trail.

I pulled out a Go Bar, my favoured protein and energy bar, and ruminated, chewing slowly. I had only come around 30 miles / 50 kilometres since the beginning of the race, but I had of course come a whole lot further than the lady in purple that nodded as she passed me just at that moment, looking irritatingly perky.

I did not have any stomach issues as I did in the Western States, and had combated cumulative fatigue in other ultras such as the Marathon Des Sables, so in that sense my situation was familiar territory. The terrain was even relatively benign, at that current moment, being around three miles / five kilometres of gently undulating cinder trail, and then a long descent to Breil.

It would be so easy to give up. To just give my bib to another runner passing, and tell them to send a Land Rover to come and get me from Breil. But I thought about Alice, and her journey. She would never have the option to throw in the towel from Diabetes, no matter how many times she said she was going to ignore the condition. She needed to treat herself and manage the condition on a daily basis. Set the alarm no matter how tired she was and check her blood sugars.

I put my pack back on, stuffing the Go Bar wrapper into a pocket, and concentrated on putting one foot in front of the other. I would just get to Breil and see how I felt.

30 June 2013, Western States 100

I had had enough. The night had gone on forever. I had rolled my ankle twice, and the strapping I had applied before the start for a slight sprain in training a couple of weeks before was the only thing holding me together.

Worse than that I had the most appalling stomach ache. I was trying to take Coke to calm it down at every aid station, but a combination of bloating and wracking hiccups prevented me from taking too much of anything in. Even an antacid gifted from a volunteer had not done anything to help me. I was staggering along the mountain path looking and sounding like I had spent all night drinking vodka in a club.

The mind plays tricks on you when you are on the trail, alone, after 80 odd miles, and I started seeing animals on the side of the trail which would look like a bear or cougar, but then dissipated as I came closer. It would turn out to be just an amalgam of bushes from the wrong angle. Then I saw two reflective studs in a tree highlighted by my headlamp. I dismissed them as trail markers, but they seemed to track me. I stopped and looked, and something cat like with big ears looked back at me. Maybe it was intrigued by my hiccups! Having read about runners on the trail being mauled and people even killed by mountain lions, I didn't hang around to introduce myself.

And then it was light. The pain from the hiccups and ankle forgotten, I packed away my headlamp, and tried to jog a little. For the first time in hours I could hear a faint hum of a car engine fading in and out, and as I continued putting one foot in front of the other, I could hear music. And then shouting. Suddenly I emerged from the path onto a road, Highway 49.

Momentum causing me to lurch, I tried to understand what the marshal was telling me about crossing it as he stopped cars to allow me to pass, and I tried to follow his pointing. I must have looked like a zombie, hollow eyed, unblinking, expressionless, covered in dirt and sweat, my formally pristine white t-shirt a nice shade of vomit yellow.

I staggered into the aid station like a drunk, where Mrs R was waiting. A sight for sore eyes. She had tried to nap in the car having arrived a few hours earlier, but had been woken by the tannoy repeatedly; as every runner came in, the announcer went ballistic with excitement. I was weighed, and although had lost weight I was about 90 miles / 144 kilometres into the race so it was to be expected to burn a little spare fat.

A few encouraging words from Mrs R, sun lotion on any exposed skin (at her prompting and despite my denials, she turned my cap around and put my sunglasses tenderly on my face). She pushed me in the direction of the exit. I was like a pliant toddler, not having the energy to argue or make any sort of decision.

I climbed out the aid station, and after a kilometre or so felt like I had wandered into an episode of *Little House On The Prairie*. The path tracked glorious parkland, reminiscent of my Kentish upbringing. Massive ancient trees broke up the plain, and a carpet of wildflowers either side of the path in all shades of purple and blue. I vividly remember watching the opening scenes of the television show with my sister as a tiny kid, with a carefree Laura running down a hill exactly the same as the one I was on. I emulated her, although minus the flowing dress, clean body, and blond plaits.

My spirits lifted from singing the theme tune to a show I had long since forgotten to myself, out loud and at full volume, I reached No Hands Bridge and overtook three or four other runners and crew, all of whom were only just perambulatory. The odd spectator was also in attendance, giving words of encouragement as I passed, and as I left the bridge I saw a familiar face.....

"Congratulations!" he said as I passed him. I couldn't quite place his face. Perhaps we had met earlier in the race, at an aid station, or at check in.

"Thanks, but I haven't finished yet," I offered back, dredging the recesses of my mind as to how I knew him. I couldn't work out where I had met him before, and then he was gone, searching out someone he knew, and I was on my never ending journey to Auburn.

"Yay Ben, well DONE! Come on!"

I looked up from watching my feet, my hands on my knees helping my legs make the final steep climb up the dirt track to Auburn.

I saw Elke as the path became paved road, and Chloe a few feet behind. They cheered when I recognised them, and to my surprise they turned around and accompanied me on my journey up the hill. They had come out to see me; me - who'd been a perfect stranger until the previous day.

Choked, I let them chat to me as I concentrated on getting to the finish.

"Did you see Tim?" Elke asked.

"Tim Twietmeyer?" she clarified, in response to my blank look.

Of course, that was where I recognised him from. Tim Twietmeyer was a local ultrarunner, and something of a legend with twenty five sub 24 hour Western States finishes to his name.[8] I had seen his picture in magazines and on the internet.

"We told him to say "hi" when he saw you. We've been tracking you all night."

I was momentarily overcome at their generosity. Not to mentioned the fact that they had adopted me as *their* runner.

The sun was already beating down, but the sights and sounds as we came into civilisation provided a welcome distraction. The road had been spray painted with directions for the runners, arrows pointing out key junctions, but both Chloe and Elke knew the way. I

---

[8] You can read more about Tim's formidable achievements with a simple google search, or here https://en.wikipedia.org/wiki/Tim_Twietmeyer

laughed as I spotted a completely drunk man with a huge beard and cool box full of beer sitting astride the sloping roof of his porch, a beat box playing heavy metal music at full volume. He cheered as we passed.

And then at the crest of the hill was Mrs R. She had changed into jogging pants and top for the last leg of the race, in order to accompany me to the finish. She could have run wearing high heels and kept up with me as my speed was not impressive. All of a sudden the tarmac gave way to running track, and there was only 400 metres left. The announcer on the tannoy was kept busy with a flurry of finishers. In the application form there was a little "Bio" section for applicants to note down a brief history, marital status, hobbies or anything else noteworthy. The announcer would then read this as the runner did a lap of the track before the finish line. It was my turn and he read out the names of my kids as Mrs R and I ran to the finish to cross the line together.

It was over. The kindness of my new friends was not, however. Elke insisted we go back to her house for a shower and celebratory beer, even though it was only 9.30am, to get ready for the medal and belt buckle presentation later that day.

1 September 2013, Ultra Trail of Mont Blanc

There comes a point in every ultra marathon where you question what you are doing, and whether you can carry on. The UTMB was no different.

Well, no; that is not true. The UTMB was like no other race.

And I had already had several of those moments during the race. I had covered about 140km of the 168km / 90 out of 105 miles; it was around 4am on the Sunday morning . I had set off at 4pm on the Friday before and been in constant motion ever since, and I was not having the moment. Someone else was.

"It looks horrendous."

"I know that. I'm looking at it. It is right in front of me."

"But how are you going to do that? It doesn't look possible."

"Darling, you're not helping here."

"But you've already scaled eight massive climbs, and this one looks the worst of the bunch. And you're exhausted."

Just at that moment I caught sight of someone hiding in the bushes. I turned to face them. They were holding a massive machine gun which was pointed at me. And were completely naked. And then, just like that, the apparition disappeared to morph into a hedge lining the path alongside a rushing river. It was cold and dark and I was exhausted. My mind was playing tricks on me, and had been for a while.

For some reason a lot of the hallucinations I was experiencing involved nudity, but I didn't have the time or energy to examine the reasons behind that, at that particular moment. I was trying to persuade Mrs R that I was going to continue the race no matter what. I had one more climb to go, over 1000m / 3000 feet of vertical, and then it was all downhill to the finish. I had plenty of time in hand, it was just a question of getting it done.

Mrs R had enjoyed the whole Western States experience so much that she had encouraged me to take up the offer of a place in the full UTMB. I had unfinished business from the previous year's shortened course, and needed to give it a go. I thought I might be able to carry some fitness from the Western States, and we had brought the kids along to help Mrs R "crew".

True to form, they had all become invested in my race. It was a real team effort with them providing moral support, bandages for a twisted ankle, homemade trail mix and powders, as well as dry clothes after a tough and damp first night. They had poured over the time logs on the race's website when trying to rest, and they were all exhausted with their efforts. Mrs R was fighting her own demons, like the little devil sitting on one shoulder telling you all the negative stuff. I took on the role of the angel on the other side and tried to boost her confidence by projecting some of my own.

"Darling, try and get some sleep. I'm just going to have to do it."

With that, I clicked off the call, then dodged a defeated runner who had given up and was coming back down the trail. I switched off my phone, and focussed on the job at hand.

20 June 2014, Cro Magnon, Breil Sur Roya

"When is it going to end?" I asked no one in particular.

After having a "moment" in the woods, I had used the old mantra "Pain is temporary. Memories are forever" to get me down the hill. Everything hurt: my feet were screaming so loud bystanders could have probably heard them; my quads were in tatters from the descents and my calves from the ascents; my lower back ached like an arthritic ninety year old's from the constant motion and back pack; my shoulders were bruised from pushing into my legs to help with the climbs, and flailing around on the descents for stability.

But most of all, I was absolutely exhausted. It wasn't like the sort of fatigue after a late night, or a broken night's sleep because of some family drama, it was deep in my bones. I had no energy. All I could focus on was getting to Breil Sur Roya for the approximate half way point to have a sit down, empty half the trail out of my shoes, and perhaps get something to eat.

A friend had made some flapjacks with oats, raisins, and honey and sent them with Mrs R to Limone. I had had quite a few after the first lap, and I had put the rest in my drop bag which would be waiting at Breil. The thought of those flapjacks was pulling me like the Star Trek tractor beam, inexorably towards them, as I salivated and hobbled.

I could hear the aid station before I could see it, as I emerged from the woods onto a paved road, and followed the river towards the music and flapjacks. Whilst the proper tarmac was playing havoc with my already destroyed feet, the thought of the moist, sweet flapjacks was keeping me going, as I imagined the constant race to get as much in my mouth as possible before they completely disintegrated.

For the first time I noticed that the light was fading. Consciously, I remembered that dusk was particularly dangerous for the mind because the body wanted to shut down ahead of a nice relaxing evening with a glass of Sauvignon Blanc and the latest Homeland episode. Subconsciously, my inner devil-voice was telling me to stop and lie down. Noone would mind. I had come so far and that was enough. My consciousness won over. Just.

I finally arrived at the checkpoint, and was met by my crew of Paola and Sonia. Paola was the aid station manager and was absolutely exhausted from the lead up to the race, as well as the long day behind her. I was four hours ahead of the cut off, as my new friends guided me to the place to pick up my drop bag and then sat me down.

I did my admin, which consisted of Vaseline application and changing the old batteries on my headlamp for some fresh ones for the fast approaching night. And then reaching for the flapjacks, whilst Sonia gabbled at me incomprehensibly in Italian.

Paola wearily translated into Franglais, and I tried to understand.

"Elle est tres bon." She's really good. "You should do it."

"Er, quoi?" What?

"Massage your legs."

"Really? I mean, is that even allowed? Ca va?"

"Sure, si, that's Sonia's job. Not just her job here, but in real life. She trained."

Happy to lose as much lactic acid as I could for the second half of my Cro, I stayed in the chair and had a glorious leg rub whilst I munched on flapjacks.

Five minutes later, I adjusted my headlamp, found the footpath in the direction of the coast, said goodbye to my friends, and marched purposefully and energetically onwards and upwards. It was like I was an old car that had had a complete bare metal respray and engine rebuild in the short space of twenty minutes.

1 September 2013, Ultra Trail of Mont Blanc
A lawnmower is not always a lawnmower...

What a climb. It was a dry glacier creek bed; glacial melt had deposited boulders and scree in the 'v' cut into the rock. There was a path with the odd step, but mainly it was scrambling over boulders and up small cliffs until a brief respite of flat. In total it was almost 1km / 625 feet of UP.

I was on the trail for my second night in a row with no sleep, and I was experiencing pain, fatigue, and bizarre thought processes that I had previously only read about. As I scaled the last climb, I tried to take my mind off the exhaustion and just focus on getting to the finish. I was reaching forwards with my hand to grip a rock and pull myself up the massive step in the hill when a fellow Brit barged past me going the other way. He had thrown in the towel, and was not alone. There would be only 1685 finishers of the 2013 UTMB out of some 2300 starters. 140 had abandoned in Courmayeur, alone, 77km / 48m into the race. As I whizzed through the aid station, it was like a scene from MASH; there must have been more than 100 people tucked up in the foetal position trying to sleep, as others applied Vaseline and bandages to various parts of their bodies.

Others caught up to me but were content to let me lead as I continued the technical climb. I was a little unsteady on my feet and given the terrain, I needed to use my hands to make sure I didn't topple over backwards. I had been hallucinating for several hours, having seen a dog that was actually a suitcase, a cat that was a discarded sweater, and bushes kept prompting my imagination to turn them into naked ladies or terrorists with assault rifles. As I climbed, hand over hand, foot over foot, I kept seeing faces in rocks; here a crocodile, built from rocks and painted; there a penguin statue; a face painted on the rock to look like the Joker from Batman. I knew that it was my exhausted mind seeing something and trying to make sense of it but coming up with the wrong answer. My consciousness was fighting my subconscious, my head trying to overrule my instinct and habit. It was strange being part of a battle that was happening inside of me.

I stopped to catch my breath at the top of the climb. Not quite dawn, but the black in the sky was giving way to an inky blue. I leaned against a plaque set on the top of the mountain, and tried to focus on the words and pictures. There was an artist in residence who had created sculptures and pictures on the climb. So not everything I had seen had been a hallucination after all.

I jogged over a few light undulations to another Col, and one of the final chip scans, where a marshall would use a hand held scanner to touch the number of every runner. Embedded in the number was a chip with each runner's details, and the rules stated that every runner had to have one; the loss of the number would result in disqualification. I had been presented with a pristine white number 905 at the expo a few days previously; 905 being my finishing rank the previous year. I had pinned it to a triathlon belt to enable the putting on and taking off of layers, and although battered, it was still present.

In the past few hours, I had discovered a dossard on the ground, muddy but still attached to an elastic belt. I looked at the flag, as each number had the runner's name and flag of nationality in each corner. It was Japanese, with an unpronounceable name.

The rules clearly stated that the loss of a number would result in a DNF, and I felt awful for that runner, because they were facing imminent disqualification. All I could do was pick it up and carry it with me in the hope I would find them at the next checkpoint. As it happened, I caught sight of a figure on the horizon and gave chase. After a few minutes I was within shouting range, and managed to squeeze out a couple of puffed "Oi!"s.

"Huh?" A Japanese man turned around with a blank look on his face.

He looked almost as exhausted as I felt.

"Have you lost your dossard?"

"No!" He insisted.

"I think you have."

"I definitely haven't. I've still got it. Look..."He looked down fully expecting to see his number on his front.

"Oh," he said. "I've lost it."

"Here." I shoved the rectangular piece of laminated cardboard into his hands, and jogged off.

I raced through the checkpoint, in reality just a couple of bored marshals in high visibility vests stamping their feet to try and keep warm. The headlamp was more of a hindrance than a help, the sky lightening with the breaking dawn, and I took it off and shoved it back into my pack. I was filled with the joy that being on the final straight brought me, the last of the ascents behind.

The ground fell away from the path and I was faced with an incredibly technical descent. I took a deep breath, turned to face the hillside and gingerly lowered myself down several "steps" in the mountain, hands and feet taking it in turns to support my weight. The going was slow, but inexorably I was getting closer to the finish.

I reached firmer ground, a sheep track with a heather border and tell-tale plastic tape marking the route. My heart sank as I saw my path blocked. How on earth was I going to get past that? On one side of the track was a steep cliff side. On the other was a long drop to the valley below. Only heather clung to the inhospitable mountain top, and years of sheep and goats making their way to fresher pastures had eaten a footpath into the terrain. In the middle of the track a lawn mower was blocking the path.

"How on earth am I going to get past that?" I said to no one in particular.

I couldn't believe it. I had come so far, about 150km / 90 miles, and was on the last descent into Chamonix and a UTMB finish, and someone had left a bloody lawn mower in the way.

"How the hell had they managed to push that up there?" I asked, knowing how heavy they were. It wasn't a riding tractor mower as that would have been too big to fit on the path. And it wasn't a cheap light electric one. It was a proper mower that they use to get the stripes just so on English cricket pitches. Maybe someone had been carting a load of rubbish for the tip along the path, and the mower had fallen off. But that didn't explain how I was going to get past.

I turned around, head down, and started back to the checkpoint. The marshals had radios, perhaps they could ask for assistance to come and move the mower.

Just then, the Japanese runner that had dropped his dossard came running down the track.

"Come on, we can finish under 40 hours. We have two hours to do the last ten kilometres," he puffed at me, and squeezed past on the narrow track.

"But how are we going to get past this lawn mower?"

"What lawn mower?" He looked at me as if I needed to be sectioned, decided not waste any more time, and charged forwards kicking up dust with each step.

I watched, intrigued as he didn't even break stride as he approached the lawn mower; and then he ran straight through it as if it wasn't even there. It was only then that I realised that the lawn mower was not real. I followed my fellow runner, although approached the blockade with a lot more trepidation than him. Sure enough, as I approached, the lawn mower disintegrated into various rocks, and I was able to pass between them as if nothing was there. Because there wasn't.

I called Mrs R, who answered the phone in a daze, and told her I was on the final descent and would be in Chamonix in an hour or two. The online predictor said I would be finishing around 40 hours and 7 minutes, but I thought that, with my latest morale boosting magic lawn mower adventure, I might be able to beat that. She promised that she and the rest of Team Rolfe would meet me at the finish.

The second sunrise of the UTMB was a subdued affair with clouds obscuring the sun, but with the dawn my

193

spirits lifted even further. I started to walk more briskly down, then jog, then run. As I approached the last Checkpoint, I was trying to overtake a chap, a sort of ultra version of the fishing game keeping my mind off the pain and fatigue and yet keeping my pace up. I could see his bib said his name was Jurgen. Trail runner etiquette states that you always let a faster person past, but he steadfastly would not let me through.

I started to get a little cross and passed through the Checkpoint, getting my chip scanned and then brushing past him while he grabbed a drink and something to nibble on.

Lost in my own thoughts about a kilometre / half a mile later, I took a wrong turn down a steep farm track, thundering down the hill into a farmyard. Realising my error, I turned and looked back at the top of the hill. Jurgen trotted past easily and laughed at my error. Trail runner etiquette demands that you yell to the person in front if you realise they are going on a wrong path and try to correct them. Jurgen had broken the rules again, which got me angry.

My blood boiled over, and I power walked back up the hill, turned back onto the right track, determined to catch, overtake, and put as much distance between myself and Jurgen before the finish. A few twists and turns, careful not to take any more wrong turns, and I could see Jurgen up ahead. I put on an extra burst as the path was flatish, meandering through some trees, and I managed to reel him in and then overtake.

The anger had helped me pick up speed and I was descending very well, despite every nerve fibre of my being screaming with pain. I was doing a lot of mental calculations to do with minutes per kilometre, how many km's I had left, and so on. I was so tired I don't think I could have done the maths even if I'd had a supercomputer with me. I just got on with it, and played the Mad Dog fishing game, putting my hook into a competitor ahead, and gradually reeling them in.

It came as a shock to emerge from the woods into Chamonix and immediately have what hardy spectators there were start to cheer me along. I tried to keep up the pace as best as I could, the tarmac harsh on my battered, blistered, exhausted feet. A right turn, and the river was on my right. I had around one kilometre left and I could see finishers, proudly sporting their finishers' gilets, hobbling along in the other direction to get to their drop bags or transport, or perhaps just lie down. I was almost there when a spectator launched into a monologue about what a great achievement I had made, and about how hard the UTMB was compared to other runs. I got a lump in my throat and a tear in my eye when I tried to mouth "Merci". I turned right again, across the river, then left into the high street, and I could see Number 1 Rolfelet waiting for me. She fell into step with me saying nothing, and we tried to sprint for the line. 200 metres later and the rest of Team Rolfe including the dog, Lucera, fell into step, and we ran the last 100 metres six abreast to great cheers.

I finished in 709th position, having overtaken 21 people in the last eight kilometres. I crossed the line in 39 hours and 48 mins, having travelled 168 km / 105m in less than two days.

People normally take two or three weeks to cover the same track.

We were all exhausted but bursting with pride at our shared achievement. The emotional investment of my family / crew was total, and they felt as mentally and physically drained, and as proud, as I did. I sat down and munched on a cold Big Mac, and some hot, sweet tea.

It was the best meal of my entire life.

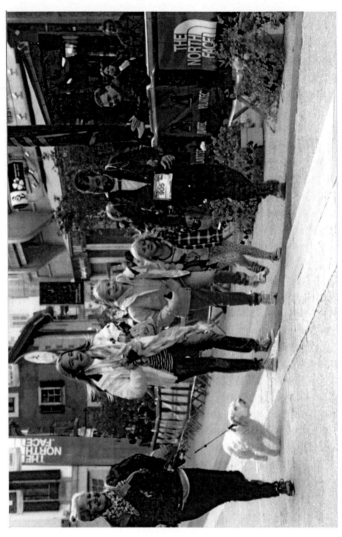

Photo by Maindru

196

20 June 2014, Cro Magnon

I left Breil singing, despite the extremely steep climb out, my morale boosted beyond compare. The path followed a nature trail etched into the hillside, with plaques detailing a specific bird or plant that could be seen in the locality. Every now and again there would be a wooden platform so as to better admire the flora and fauna and of the views as I climbed out of the valley. I even stopped to read the Wild Boar (Sanglier) plaque to find out what a baby wild boar was called, but as quickly as I added to my French vocabulary it was lost around the next corner.

Experience had taught me that dusk was going to be tricky, and I kept having to remind myself that the body was trying to shut down in readiness for a relaxing evening in front of the TV with a glass of something nice in hand. I knew that as soon as the sun disappeared below the horizon I would perk up, have more energy, and be able to tackle the long night ahead. It didn't make it any easier as the sky lost its lustre and turned grey. I had the cumulative fatigue from the race itself but also from the lost night's sleep a day or two previously on my way to Limone.

Contrary to the run in to Breil, I actually found myself keeping pace with other runners again, and occasionally overtaking them. As night fell, I crested a mountain to leave the Roya Valley, descending into the same valley I had run through a couple of days previously. Further up the river was the town of Sospel, although the route dictated a steep descent to intersect the river quite a long way downstream from Sospel.

The sun disappeared completely, and the fireflies came out to play.

The pain was overtaking the morale boosting time at the aid station, but the fireflies helped enormously. One actually landed on my sleeve, its light blinking on and off. They are surprisingly large, the luminescent bulb at the bottom of their abdomen a small portion of the creature itself. A brief pit stop and my new friend lumbered slowly off, frantically beating its wings, struggling to carry its own weight.

My headlamp was picking out clouds of dust giving a spotlight effect in my path, as I followed the footpath with the river to my left. Ducking under branches and hurdling roots, but importantly moving forwards. Eventually I could hear a party going on in Sospel, and as I emerged from the woods, the path crossed some agricultural land, and then turned into track and paved road.

I arrived in Sospel at around 10.25pm, my second visit in three days.

Or was it four? Too tired to count, or even care.

In previous iterations, the aid station had been massive with three or four tables, masseurs, cheering bystanders, and medical staff. I had managed to catch up with a couple of other runners on the last two kilometres into the village, and they had eagerly discussed having a seat and some hot pasta or soup when they arrived.

We were all disappointed to pass through a playground into the main square, which doubled as a car park, to be greeted by a couple of trestle tables offering merely Coke and water. No matter, I wasn't interested in a three course meal anyway. I did what I always do: filled my backpack with fluids, had half a Go Bar whilst cleaning out my shoes of various bits of trail debris, and then was on my way after grabbing a plastic cup of Coke.

As I trotted out the square, a couple of volunteers scanned my chip, and I managed a little joke with them, something about meeting them same time same place in a year's time.

The climb out of Sospel was brutal. I knew that from bitter experience, and I mentally prepared myself as I tried to follow the spray painted arrows on the tarmac. I knew this path well, having run it on many trail races and also run down it on my journey to the start a couple of days previously. It was no easier than I had remembered. The gradient was such that on a couple of occasions I was in danger of toppling over backwards; I had to frantically flail around until I could grab a branch or tree root to regain my balance.

Always a morale booster, I overtook a couple of guys who were struggling, and managed to navigate the path correctly despite the odd missing trail marker. One chap was stumbling back down the hill, holding on to a bush to slow his descent and the veins popping out on his calves as his legs braced themselves whilst he slid and stumbled down the path. His body appeared fit enough to carry on, but it was clear that he had given up in his head. His race was over.

I was heading for Peille, but the climb out of Sospel was seemingly never ending. Hands on knees to help the legs cope with the interminable ascent, one foot after the other. Either side of the path was thick forest, and at night was frighteningly dark. I was taking care to keep an eye on the trail markers, as one wrong turn and I would be hopelessly lost within minutes.

The endless climb, dust, dark and loneliness began to take their toll. I knew in my head it would be over after 10km / 6m and 1000 metres / 3000 feet of altitude change, and my head began to droop. I needed a boost, and called a friend that I knew would still be up at that ungodly hour. The remoteness meant the signal was weak, and we played telephone tennis for a few minutes. Thankfully Mark knew what I needed and left a joke on my answer phone. I listened to it on repeat as I finished the rest of the climb, chuckling to myself as I went.

I caught up another runner, someone I had briefly chatted to earlier in the race, and at the top we asked the marshal how much further to Peille. He said it was a 7km / 4m descent, which was music to our ears. Peille was a village a little behind the coast. From there it did not seem very far at all to the finish.

After a couple of kilometres my new friend started to wobble and weave like a drunk leaving a nightclub. I put my arm around his waist and tried to help him by pointing out how far we had gone and how it was not much further to Peille, but he was too far gone. He stopped, and as we emerged onto a paved road, he sat down in the middle of the road, and started to go to sleep using his back pack as a pillow.

I was pretty sure it was just fatigue, but even if it was, the ambient temperature once stationary was not ideally suited to having a nap, especially as he was wearing three quarter length Lycra trousers and a thin rainproof jacket. I did my best to move him off the road should a car come, fending off his half asleep protestations. It was only a single lane path, probably some sort of farm or national park track and I didn't realistically expect any traffic passing, at least not until morning. Another runner passed by focussed on his own race, as I was reaching for my mobile to call for help. No signal. Bugger.

But I could hear voices, faint but distinct, a bit further down the path. I thought perhaps the passing runner had met someone else on the trail, someone who could help. I left the runner to his nap, checking he was still breathing, and ran down the hill as fast as my exhausted body would carry me. Only a couple of hundred metres later and I encountered a volunteer medical team of three. I quickly explained the situation, and left them to trek up with their first aid kits.

I raced on knowing that they would be with him in a few short minutes.

In mountain ultra trail races, I had come to learn that a marshal's perception of a kilometre or mile wasn't necessarily the same as a participant's. The same went for descents. The descent into Peille became an evil little climb just before reaching the village. A morale and energy sapping thirty minutes later, I reached the second-to-last checkpoint of the race.

I changed the batteries in my headtorch, and was grateful for a cup of tea with a sugar lump to warm me. I had built up a sizeable margin to finish within the cut off time, and could afford a short sit down whilst I dealt with my admin. It was very tempting to sit there and perhaps have a short nap. The aid station was in some sort of village hall, and was packed with runners and bleary eyed volunteers and their kids, milling around, with seats in great demand. It was a useful reminder to get moving again when another runner staggered through the door a few minutes after me looking for somewhere to rest.

I grabbed a Coke chaser for my tea, topped off the fluids in my pack, and left the hubbub of the checkpoint, knowing without a doubt that I was going to finish. It was a short distance to the final ridge and from there I knew every footpath down to the finish like the back of my hand.

I was practically in my own back yard.

The route up to the Col de Madone was as technical as ever, a very steep climb through a wood to the windblown radar station at the top. I passed a couple, woman and man, arguing in Italian, as I went. The Cro Magnon had to have been a true test of their relationship and I silently wished them all the best as I passed.

I was pleasantly surprised we hadn't been sent up to the very top of the Col, as about two thirds of the way up we veered back down the hill and I could see the twinkling lights of Monaco and the Riviera below me. The moon was shining on the rippling Med, and I took a moment to enjoy the view. I was on the final "straight" and I felt like I was sprinting.

Passing the Monte Carlo Golf Club as dawn was just starting to raise its head, I overtook quite a few more people employing the fishing game, reeling in competitors as I went. I called Mrs R and Mark H and said it would be around an hour and a half until the finish, depending on the route. As the crow flies I could have covered the ground in about thirty minutes, but sure enough, just before La Turbie and the final check point we were sent off to do another climb and descent before we arrived at the aid station. I bet Pietro and the organisers got a little chuckle at that one.

The last aid station was La Turbie. I got my ticket scanned and refused all food and drinks, barely even slowing down. I was nearly done.

The Brit I had met earlier in the race and an Italian he had been running with for most of the race joined me, in as much of a rush as me. I led them through La Turbie and onto the Tete de Chien track for the descent to the finish. They set off apace, but I had to stop. I was momentarily breathless. I put my hands on my knees just as the sun breached the horizon to my left, and I gasped for breath like a fish out of water. I had no energy at all.

Gradually I was able to regain my composure, and I took a few slurps of my electrolyte drink. Keeping up with my companions was out of the question; I had to make my own way home. I walked slowly for a hundred metres, then was able to jog a little, and as the course took a very sharp left to switchback down the mountain I started to skip over rocks and boulders strewn on the narrow track.

I overtook one, then another as I zig zagged down the path, and then through the streets of Cap D'Ail. I could taste the salt from the sea as I jogged onto the Sentier Littoral which ran alongside the sea, and I ran as fast as I could, knowing my family would be waiting for me at the finish.

Running into the sun, I heard rather than saw them, as I turned the final corner, and my hands were grabbed by my eldest daughters, Emily and Alice; we sprinted onto the stony beach to cross the red carpet and to finish.

Pietro and I embraced with tears in our eyes as the enormity of the achievement washed over us. As soon as I had composed myself, the Master of Ceremonies asked me to say a few words about what I had done and what I was doing it for. I managed a few words in French about Diabetes and thanked everyone, but my body was creaking. As soon as I had finished, I hobbled the last ten yards to the sea, shucked off my pack and shoes, and waded into the Mediterranean fully clothed. Mrs R threw me a sandwich and a Coke as I sat there letting my legs, still twitching, be caressed by the velvet-like water.

The hours and days after the event seemed rather surreal. Ten years prior I had considered, rightly, completing a marathon to be a massive achievement. Several years later I had completed two in a year, and now two in one go!

To have covered 235km / 147 miles, 12800m / 38000 feet of up and the same down, and almost three nights of no sleep was a feat that I still struggle to comprehend. A total of forty one and a half hours of motion in three and a half days over some of the toughest terrain in the world.

My feet were restricted to espadrilles for a week, but the profile of Diabetes and the monies we raised made it all worthwhile.

I had also proven to myself and my daughters that anything is possible if we are determined enough to succeed. No matter the obstacles in the way.

Never one to look back, I thought to myself, what next?

18 March 2015, Home to Homeland 5.50pm

Just as I was putting on my jacket and getting ready to head home after a slow day at the office, the bell sounded on my pc, indicating a client had sent me an instant message. The markets had closed fifteen minutes before, and most of the guys in the office had already gone, some headed home or to the gym, but a large contingency heading to the cinema to watch one of the few showings of the latest blockbuster in English.

The client wanted to do a trade. It was not something that could be executed in the market; he wanted to arbitrage the difference between a UK listed entity and the Australian listing of the same company. It also required a foreign exchange transaction, and then a complicated booking process. I quickly hit speed dial to one of the counterparties that could be counted on to facilitate the transaction, and within a few seconds had lined up the other side.

A little to-ing and fro-ing between the clients with some negotiating, and eventually I was able to match a price and terms, and I crossed the trade between the two. I had to then work out the numbers on the foreign exchange transaction, and agree with one of the counterparties on the exact moment we hit the "Trade" button on our trading screens to avoid paying more than the bid offer spread (which would mean giving up some of our profit).

Entering all the parameters into my spreadsheet, I went through the laborious booking process. Fortunately, in the end everything worked out and the commission on the trade made it worth going into the office that day; I headed home with a spring in my step.

6.50pm

"Isabelle, where is your English book?" I heard Mrs R asking, in a marginally exasperated voice, as I walked through the door and was greeted by two bouncing balls of white fluff demanding my attention.

"Bwoah." Answered Izzy, in the parlance of the day, meaning "I dunno", but without actually moving her lips and seemingly designed to annoy any parents within 50 paces.

"Look up from your iPod when I'm speaking to you," Mrs R said, in a slightly more elevated tone.

I unzipped my coat and turned into the kitchen; amidst the clouds of steam from stirring three saucepans, Mrs R was simultaneously looking at Izzy's homework book.

"Hi darling, how..." I managed to get out.

"Dogs need a walk," she said to me without looking up, still trying to decipher Izzy's handwriting and work out how she was going to tackle the evening's homework without the necessary books at home.

As I exited the kitchen, Alice came charging down the stairs and barged past me. "MUM! WHY AM I SO HIGH ALL THE TIME?" She screamed, flounced round the kitchen and then slumped on the floor near the dogs' water bowl.

"What's happened?" Mrs R and I both asked simultaneously.

"Bwoah," said Alice, shrugging in an altogether Gallic fashion.

"Alice how can we help if you won't give us any information?" We both responded.

"Oh for God's sake. I don't know," Alice responded. "I was 10 after I came home from school and now I'm 14. What's wrong with me? I hate it. I HATE IT! I'm not going to be diabetic any more. That's it. I'm going on strike."

"Darling, it's the pump. Let's change that." Mrs R said, as I nodded in agreement. Alice just shrugged, and slumped even more so that she was almost lying in the dogs' bowl.

A few minutes later, having gone through the rigmaroles of changing the reservoir and cannula on the pump, I left Mrs R once more wrestling with the cooking and homework, to go walk the dogs. I arrived home to the sound of Mrs R yelling through the smoke of burnt pasta at everyone and no one in particular about the unreasonable and simultaneous demands on her time from everyone. The smoke alarm went off, and I gagged, reaching for the corkscrew.

7.30pm

We eventually sat down to dinner; two different pasta sauces as Izzy refuses to eat mushrooms and Emily refuses to eat carrots or cheese; two different types of slightly crispy ravioli as the packets are always for four, not five.

Ding. Mrs R's phone.

"What's that?" I asked.

"Isabelle's homework," she replied.

"Oh ok, that's good. Who sent it?"

"Elena's Mum."

"Dad, you have to put up a picture for me," Emily 'asked', interrupting.

"What? Now?"

"No, after supper is fine."

"But it'll be gone 8.30pm after supper. I don't want to do it then. Firstly I'm tired, and secondly the neighbours don't want to hear banging when they are trying to relax." (Ah, the joys of living in an apartment.)

"Oh for God's sake! Mum! He won't do it."

"Your Dad has a point, darling. The weekends are for DIY."

A huge angry sigh from Emily as she found a stray carrot in her food and disgustedly threw it away. She finished eating as quickly as she could, stomped up the stairs and slammed her door shut behind her.

206

8.55pm

Mrs R and I slumped onto our respective positions in the sitting room, a large glass of Bordeaux apiece. I was splayed out on the floor, slumped against a couple of cushions and pressed up against a sofa with our dog my recent addition and second dog, Jack alongside me, contentedly having his tummy rubbed. Mrs R lay on the other sofa with Lucera snuggled at her feet, snoring. I reached for the remote, and was greeted with the wonderful, discordant, disembodied dialogue of the Homeland opening credits. The recap from the previous episode was just starting. I had been looking forward to watching that episode all day. It was the last one of the Season and the previous episode had ended on a dramatic cliffhanger. No more than five seconds in, and the distinctive stomp stomp stomp of someone angrily descending the stairs. The windows rattled as the sitting room door slammed open.

Emily launched herself into the sitting room headfirst landing on the floor, narrowly missing my wine glass, sending the dogs scurrying for cover, and whispered "I feel funny." With that she closed her eyes, rolled over onto her back, arms outstretched, and lay motionless.

Mrs R and I looked at each other. I got up to find a Blood Glucose monitor, and Mrs R disappeared to the kitchen. I pricked Alice's finger, and waited for the monitor to bleep. She was just over two mmol, very low. After changing the pump, we had obviously over corrected and possibly over estimated the carbs at supper, and she was having a bad hypo, the target range being between four and six. Mrs R reappeared with a variety of dextrose tablets, fizzy drinks and biscuits, all useful for a quick boost to the Blood Glucose Level (BGL).

9.50pm

Mrs R and I slumped onto our respective positions in the sitting room, once more with a large glass of Bordeaux apiece. I was splayed out on the floor, slumped against a couple of cushions and pressed up against a sofa with Jack alongside me, contentedly having his tummy rubbed. Mrs R lay on the other sofa with Lucera snuggled at her feet, snoring. Alice's mini crisis dealt with, she had finally calmed enough to relax and hopefully go to sleep.

The recap from the previous episode was just starting. I had been looking forward to watching that episode all day. It was the last one of the Season and the previous episode had ended on a dramatic cliff hanger. No more than five seconds in, and the distinctive stomp stomp stomp of someone angrily descending the stairs. The windows rattled as the sitting room door slammed open.

"Now look what you've done!" Alice pointed at me, looking at me with tear filled eyes.

"What have I done?" I turned to Mrs R who just shrugged.

"You broke my picture!" She waved a small photo frame in my direction, little shards flying off from the broken glass.

"I never touched it!" I said defensively, having never even laid eyes on it. "I've been here the whole time. Well, apart from dealing with your sister, I mean."

"Yes, but if you'd put it up, it wouldn't have broken." The tears started to come.

Mrs R interjected. "Emily, how did the picture actually break?"

"Erm...I sat on it." She said.

10.30pm

Mrs R and I slumped onto our respective positions in the sitting room, a large glass of Bordeaux apiece. I was splayed out on the floor, slumped against a couple of cushions and pressed up against a sofa with Jack alongside me, contentedly having his tummy rubbed. Mrs R lay on the other sofa with Lucera snuggled at her feet, snoring. The recap from the previous episode of Homeland was just starting. I had been looking forward to watching that episode all day. It was the last one of the Season and the previous episode had ended on a dramatic cliff hanger.

I glanced over to check my running kit was laid out behind me, ready for the early morning alarm to go off. I blinked a couple of times, each one more protracted than the last, and the last thing I saw was Carrie Matthews about to deliver the first line of the episode, before falling asleep.

Lightning Source UK Ltd.
Milton Keynes UK
UKOW02f1417230516

274827UK00001B/1/P